D0688224

Alive with Alzheimer's

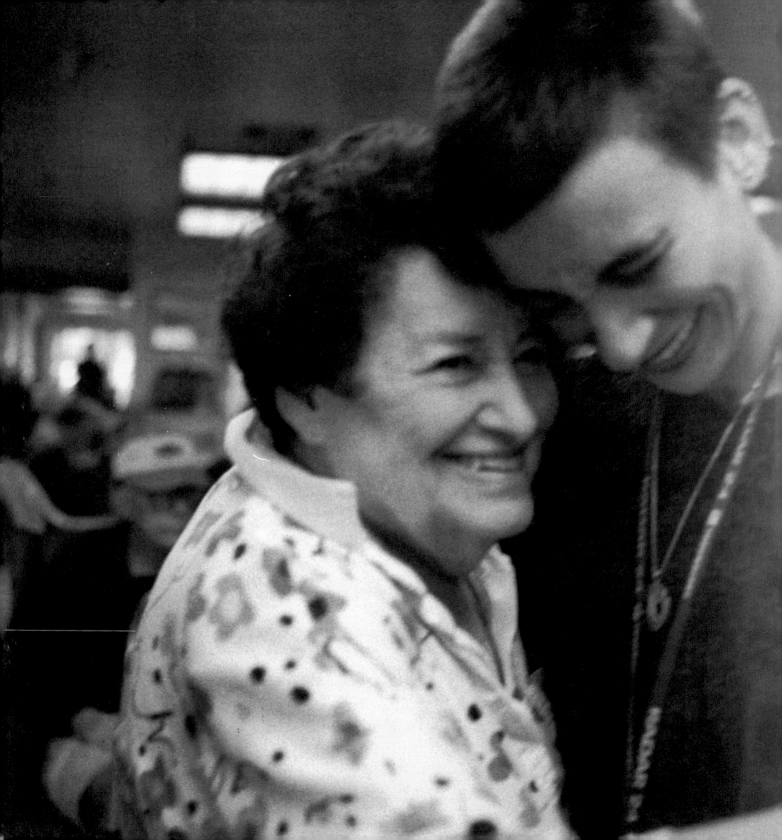

Alive with Alzheimer's

Cathy Stein Greenblat

The University of Chicago Press
Chicago and London

Cathy Stein Greenblat is Professor Emerita at Rutgers University, where she was a member
of the Department of Sociology, the Women's Studies faculty, and the faculty of the Edward
Bloustein School of Planning for more than thirty-five years. Among her previous books
are *The Marriage Game; Getting Married; Life Designs; Designing Games and Simulations;* and
Principles and Practices of Gaming-Simulation. She has lectured around the world and has
exhibited her photography in the United States, Europe, Asia, and the Middle East.

The University of Chicago Press, Chicago 60637
The University of Chicago Press, Ltd., London
© 2004 by The University of Chicago
Photographs © 2004 by Cathy Stein Greenblat
All rights reserved. Published 2004
Printed in the United States of America

13 12 11 10 09 08 07 06 05 04   1 2 3 4 5
ISBN: 0-226-30658-5 (cloth)

Library of Congress Cataloging-in-Publication Data
Greenblat, Cathy S., 1940–
     Alive with Alzheimer's / Cathy Stein Greenblat.
        p. cm.
     Includes bibliographical references.
     ISBN 0-226-30658-5 (cloth : alk. paper)
     1. Alzheimer's disease—Patients—Long-term care. 2. Alzheimer's disease—
Patients—Pictorial works. 3. Alzheimer's disease—Long-term care—California—
Escondido. 4. Alzheimer's disease—Long-term care—California—Escondido—Pictorial
works. [DNLM: 1. Alzheimer Disease—Pictorial Works. WT 17 G798a 2004] I. Title.
RC523 .G745 2004
362.196′831′00222—dc22

                                              2003016073

This book is printed on acid-free paper.

For John H. Gagnon,
who always helps me remember what is important

Poem Sent on a Sheet of Paper with a Heart Shape Cut Out of
the Middle of It

Empty or open-hearted? Where
A full heart spoke once, now a strong
Outline is the most I dare:
A window opening onto fair
Shining meadows of hopefulness? Or long
Silence where there once was song,
Waves of remembrance in the darkening air.

—John Hollander

Contents

1

Facing Alzheimer's

IN THE MID-1960S, I lost my maternal grandfather. He died four years later. The official diagnosis was "hardening of the arteries." Initially, he was "confused," disoriented, and paranoid about money; later, he often became angry and physically resistant to requests. Finally, he began to wander around the neighborhood in his pajamas in the middle of the night.

Unable to care for him anymore, even with the help of a live-in nurse, my grandmother made the difficult decision to place him in an institution—the best one she could find. He had pleasant nurses, a clean room, and medications that kept him from making problems for the staff. Occasionally restraints were used when he was particularly agitated and difficult. He spent his last two years of life there.

My grandmother visited daily; my mother visited weekly. He was pleased to see them but distressed at how they looked: he had lost his short-term memory, and he thought they were twenty years younger. "Why do you have so many gray hairs and wrinkles?" he asked.

I was in my mid-twenties. I cried for a week after my first visit to the nursing home. Poppy had raged that I was an impostor, not his granddaughter. "Cathy is a child, and you are a woman. . . . Don't tell me you're my granddaughter. . . . You are just another person trying to cheat me out of my hard-earned money!" The only way I could visit him after that was to deny that we were grandfather and granddaughter. I had to pretend to be just a friendly visitor. He was then warm and talkative, but I was paralyzed, unable to handle the situation well.

Poppy had been a brilliant, successful trial attorney. A family story often told to me was that Governor Dewey, had he become President Dewey, intended to name my grandfather to the U.S. Supreme Court. Throughout my childhood Poppy visited our home regularly, talking to me at length about his latest victory in court and the latest triumph of his beloved Brooklyn Dodgers. I dreamed of becoming a lawyer, and I learned all the statistics for my team, the New York Yankees. We battled every Sunday to see who knew the most about their team. He encouraged my success in school and told me that a girl "could" become a lawyer if she really wanted to and worked hard.

Poppy never left the nursing home after he was placed there, except to go to the hospital when he broke his hip. On my rare visits I would ask him how he was. Each time, he told me about the case he was trying in court and about the baseball game he had attended the day before. The details of the case were identical to those I had heard two decades earlier when he was actively practicing. The details of the game were equally accurate—there were pitchers and runs and double plays I could recall from our days together at World Series games (often featuring the Yankees versus the Dodgers in those years).

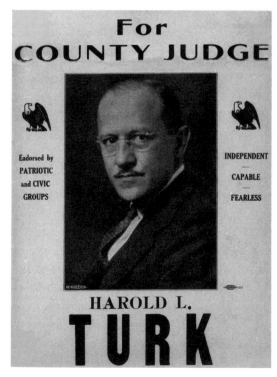

"Poppy," September 21, 1893–May 1, 1968

No one helped me handle my emotional turmoil, and eventually I stopped visiting my grandfather. I also stopped thinking about going to law school, and I stopped watching baseball games.

Today my grandfather would be diagnosed as having Alzheimer's disease, that progressive, degenerative disease of the brain, which is the most common form of dementia. There would still be no cure, and his medical treatment would not be much different, though an early diagnosis might delay the onset of more problematic symptoms. My grandmother would resist placing him in an institutional setting, where Alzheimer's patients still are often highly medicated and often restrained. Such a placement would be a last resort, when Alzheimer's became too much for the family setting. My grandfather would be living with Alzheimer's but not alive with it.

In the summer of 2001, having been an academic sociologist for several decades, I spent six weeks photographing at Silverado Senior Living, a specialized residential care facility in Escondido, California, for people with Alzheimer's and other forms of dementia. I found Silverado almost by accident, through a network of sympathetic acquaintances who had seen my earlier photographs taken in a Mexican municipal old-age home. I had told them I was looking for a place to expand my body of photographic work on aging.

All the ninety Silverado residents had significant short-term memory loss, and those in more advanced stages of their illness had lost much of their long-term memory as well. All of them were often confused and disoriented and subject to dramatic mood shifts. They had difficulty finding the right words to express themselves. There were long silences. They had become strangers to their pasts.

From my first visit, I sensed that Silverado offered a care environment, philosophy, and practice that was radically different from what I had seen as a young adult visiting my grandfather in his nursing home. It also contrasted sharply with what I knew from my casual reading about Alzheimer's treatment. I wanted to know more about Silverado, and I decided to use my photographic skills and my sociological perspective to explore and document this place.

It was time for me to face Alzheimer's yet again. After my grandfather's death in 1969, my grandmother had developed the disease and spent her final ten years in a nursing home. She did not speak for the last four years, from the time she was 90 until she died in the mid-1980s at age 94. My mother had had a series of strokes in 1998 and was suffering from multi-infarct dementia. Her doctor thought she was also showing signs of early stage Alzheimer's. I have studied statistics, and I know how to assess probabilities. My chances of avoiding this fate are not good. A field work project at Silverado, I felt, might help me face my own fears.

The residents at Silverado are spouses, parents, and grandparents who have been placed there by their families. Usually this exceedingly difficult and painful decision is made after the Alzheimer's sufferer has begun to wander from home, has lost the ability to care for himself or herself, and is angered or frightened by family members, who have become strangers. Some of the people I spoke with had visited dozens of facilities before placing their family member at Silverado. One woman had moved across the country with her mother, finding a new job and a new home near the facility. Others commuted on a regular basis from Toronto, New York, or Atlanta to visit. "We didn't find anything like this near us," they told me.

Currently about 4 million Americans and 15 million people worldwide have been diagnosed with Alzheimer's disease. Given the persisting popular belief that senility is a normal part of aging, not the result of a disease, the number of diagnoses probably severely underestimates the number of cases. While there is always the hope that medical research will yield a solution, current estimates are that the situation will become worse in the near future. According to Zaven Khachaturian, director of the Alzheimer's Association Ronald and Nancy Reagan Research Institute, "The numbers are going to double every twenty years. Not only that: The duration of illness is going to get much longer. There's the really devastating part. The folks who have the disease now are mostly people who came through the depression. Some had a college education, but most did not. The ones who are going to develop Alzheimer's in the next century will be baby boomers who are primarily better educated and much better fed. The duration of their disability is going to be much longer" (quoted in Shenk 2001, p. 61). Many people, then, must learn to face the possibility of Alzheimer's affecting themselves or their loved ones. Yet many avoid thinking about it and consequently risk being as incompetent at dealing with their loved ones as I was with my grandfather and my grandmother.

My training and my professional career have been in sociology; my research methods of choice have been ethnography (field work) and visual sociology (a way of integrating visual imagery into the research process). Ethnographers spend considerable time at a site, suspending assumptions, gathering data through observation and intensive interviews, organizing that data, and presenting ideas. Visual sociologists photograph not only to have an aide-mémoire as they review their notes, but also to present elements of their findings in a way that could not be offered as effectively through words.

This book is the result of such an investigation. I spent many weeks at Silverado, observing, conversing with residents, staff, and family members, and taking part in some activities. I also sat in on family support group sessions led by Dr. Enid Rockwell, a geriatric psychiatrist. Mostly, however, I photographed, taking more than one thousand photos in all. I present here only a small portion of what I saw. I offer an interpretation of what I feel to be the key elements of a care process that provides a view of Alzheimer's patients that is different from what most of us know and from what is generally found in popular and scholarly literature.

The photographs are, for me, the key element, but they do not speak entirely for themselves. I have therefore added some of my own thoughts and excerpts from interviews with staff members and family members. Some of these conversations were what visual sociologists refer to as "photo elicitation interviews." I showed people stacks of photographs, and they talked with me about what they thought and felt while looking through them. Unfortunately, few of the residents had enough cognitive functioning to be interviewed in the conventional sense, though I had warm exchanges with many of them. The photographs must substitute for their words.

I worked to document a particular place in the hope that the results might illuminate larger personal and policy issues in Alzheimer's care. This goal is consistent with the aims expressed by documentary photographer Mary Ellen Mark: "What I'm trying to do is to make photographs that are universally understood, whether in China or Russia or America—photographs that cross cultural lines. . . . If it's about famine in Ethiopia, it's about the human condition all over the world: it's about people dying in the streets of New York as much as it's about Ethiopia. I want my photographs to be about the basic emotions and feelings that we all experience" (Mark 1990, pp. 9–10).

The visual dimension of infirmity and death is frightening. We avert our gaze. As private photographers documenting important moments in our lives, we avoid the subjects of illness and death. We photograph birthdays, weddings, anniversaries, and family reunions, focusing on those who are on their best behavior, not on those who are quarreling, fighting, drunk, disorderly, or miserable. And we do not photograph our loved ones at times of illness, accidents, funerals, wakes, or during the grieving process following a death.

Professional photographers sometimes deal with illness and death, but in the public sphere. They show us images of dramatic moments of death and suffering associated with human tragedies of famine, accidents, crimes, epidemics, and war. The work of Eric Heider, Gilles Peress, and Sebastian Salgado are excellent examples of this type of photography. Yet Richard Avedon was accused of exploiting his father's illness for his own career ends when he published stark images of his father during the last months of his life.

Avedon is not the only photographer to have explored the private realm, however, and I have been moved and instructed by the following photographic projects on everyday illness and death: Dan and Mark Jury's beautiful small volume, *Gramp*, touched me greatly. Young photographers when their beloved grandfather developed what would today be identified as Alzheimer's disease, they used their cameras to document his decline and passing. The book is tender and full of sweetness. Martine Franck offers fine images of the aging process in *Un temps de vieillir* . . . Matt Rainey and Robin Gary Fisher won a 2001 Pulitzer Prize for their eight-month documentation of the plight and partial recovery of burn victims from the Seton Hall University dormitory fire (Rainey and Fisher 2000; Markisz 2001). Marrie Bot's beautiful book *Bezwaard Bestaan*, published in the Netherlands, sensitively illustrates and discusses the problems of those with physical disabilities, showing those who are often thought of as "funny" and "strange" to be warm, human beings. Jo Spence's writings about photographic imagery of disability are all thought provoking.

Current discussions of people with Alzheimer's are full of the language of death: "Mother is not the person we knew—that person died"; "at the nursing home I saw people who are totally gone"; "the first death was when I placed her in an institution, and the second was when she actually passed away." My outlook before I undertook this project, indeed the way I described the loss of my grandfather above, accords with these feelings. The few photographs I have seen of people with Alzheimer's also highlight the "dead" elements of their state.

My view has changed. While I concur that the ravages of Alzheimer's disease are devastating to the individual with the disease and to family members, as they were and are to me, I have witnessed another, parallel reality, one that challenges our stereotypes and defies conventional approaches to Alzheimer's care. I hope I can help the readers of this book witness it, too. Although people with Alzheimer's have lost some of the characteristics that their friends and family treasured, they are still capable of living and loving, and they are in need of and responsive to loving attention in return. My hope is that these photographs from Silverado will show that this loving attention can occur in an institutional setting, that there are things that can be done to allow people with Alzheimer's to remain *alive*, not just living with the disease. In learning this lesson, patients, families, and staff members of other Alzheimer's treatment facilities will be enriched. And maybe we will all be less fearful about our own futures.

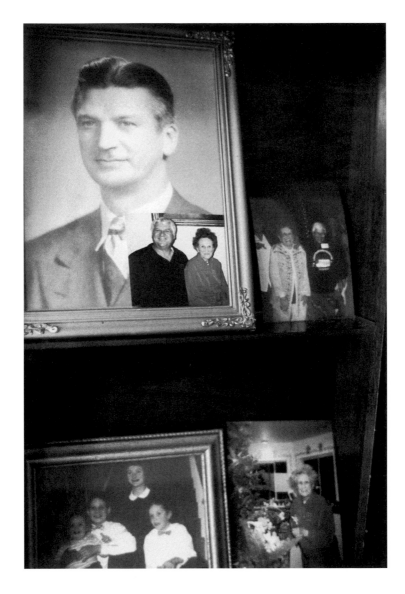

"Memory boxes" in the hall contain photographs and memorabilia.
These help residents to locate their rooms, for they often recognize items in it
or images of loved ones from earlier years.

2

Long Silence Where There Once Was Song

HILDA WAS LOST AGAIN. She asked me for help.

"Where is the bathroom? I have to wee-wee."
"Where is my room?"
"Did we have dinner yet? Will you eat with me?"

Hilda is not, as you might have imagined, a small child. She is a ninety-year-old woman with severe memory loss due to Alzheimer's disease.

Some of Hilda's other questions were also easy to answer:

"Is my husband still alive?" "No."
"Do I have children?"
"Yes, and they come to visit you whenever they can."

But I never knew how to answer the question that sometimes appeared in her eyes, which seemed to inquire, "Who am I?"

I felt this most acutely the day Hilda asked me to accompany her to the beauty parlor. She looked so much older than she had at other times. I later saw that it was common for the residents of Silverado to show significant changes in expression and in general appearance from one hour to the next. The extent of these changes was sometimes dismaying.

Hilda did not usually remember who I was from one visit to the next, but I had become a familiar friendly face and voice. One day I had spent about an hour chatting with her and photographing her. She was full of warmth, but it was hard to capture her softness because she had lost most of her subcutaneous tissue. As we sat together for cookies and juice, she asked another question:

"Will you be my friend?"
"Absolutely. I would like that very much."
"Then I won't be so lonely."

We concluded the deal with a hug, and we both were less alone and less lost.

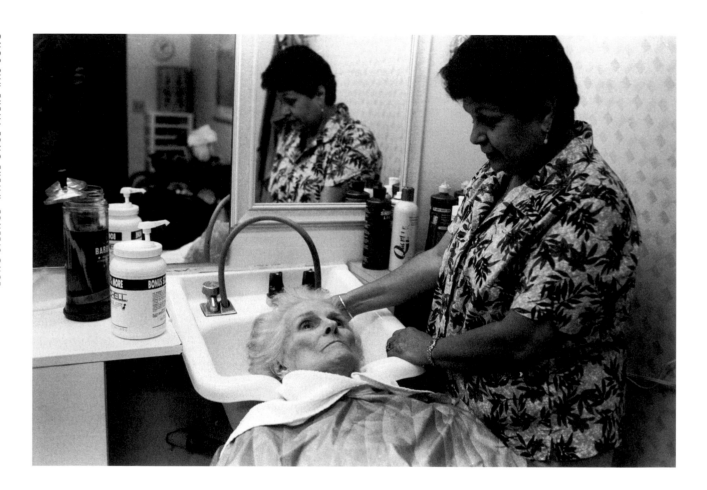

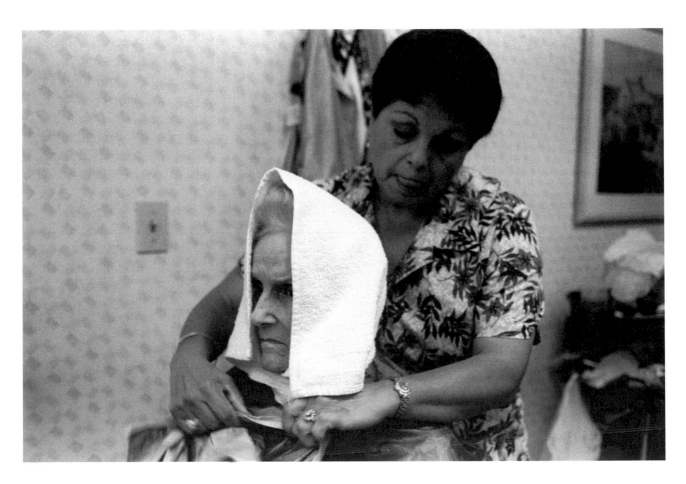

Hilda's usual good spirits were not evident the day I accompanied her to the beauty parlor.

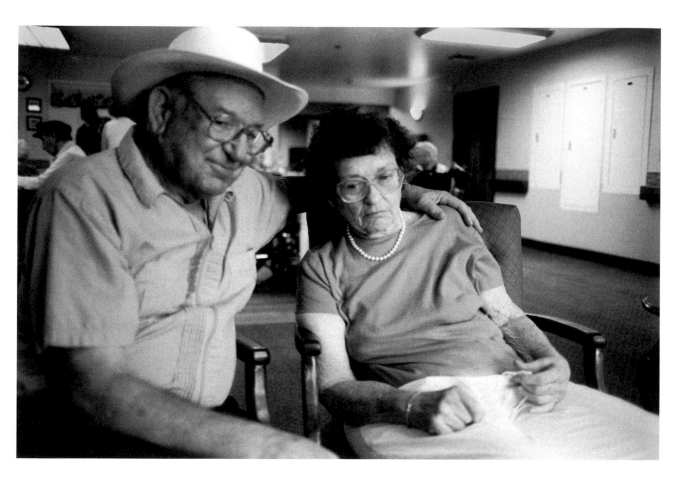

Liz knew that Ken was a friendly person who came to visit her every day. Only rarely did she recognize him
as the devoted husband who cared for her at home during the first ten years of her illness,
and who turned her care over to others with great hesitation. In the rare moments that
Liz showed she recognized Ken or something he said, his eyes filled with delight.

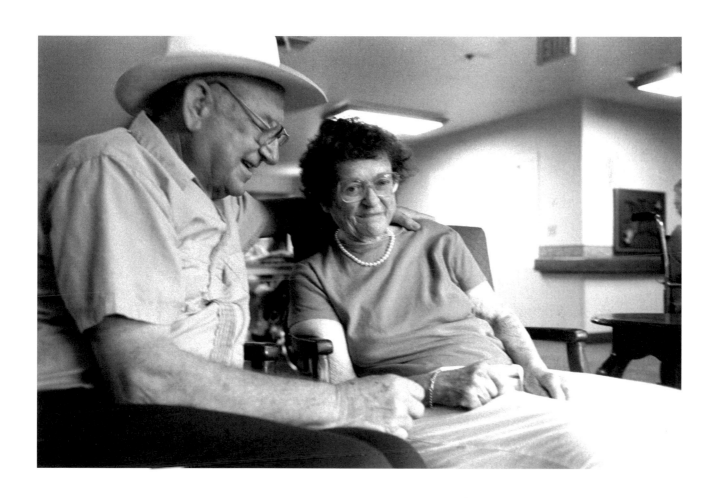

Igor had a doctorate in the physical sciences and
held many patents. At the time I photographed him,
he no longer remembered the skills with which he had achieved
eminence in his field. Since his arrival at Silverado, a year and
a half before my field work, he had been taken off psychotropic
medicines completely, and his family felt his stay was successful.
But the disease progressed, and I saw that he frequently
looked as lost when his loving wife and son were present as
he looked when they were absent. Clearly, however, he was happy
when they came to see him.

A caregiver on the staff, looking at the photographs on pages
13 and 14, commented as follows:

"This is a very dedicated family. Igor is very proud of his son,
even though he sometimes doesn't recognize him.
I see that Igor is rather distant here; he's not really enveloped
in the conversation. Igor is such a brilliant man,
he must be thinking, 'Where are the words, where are the
thoughts?' Or maybe he's just happy to be there, idle and quiet,
I don't know. But he does have his son's support.
Igor's thoughts come and go, and usually he livens up again
through a cup of tea.

"His son is concerned, watching his father and looking for
a way to establish communication with him. It must be hard to
see his father in this state, but I know that he makes his father
as happy as he can while he's here. When you see them
together now, you can tell that his father showed a lot of
compassion to his son earlier in his life.

"Igor and his wife are so dedicated—they're so in love with
each other. When his family comes, his eyes light up, his blue eyes
that show so much emotion. She brings some sweets,
like cookies, each time she comes. She always brings something
to show she cares, something he remembers.

"He's a brilliant man, and he's such a wonderful character.
He's in his own world right now. I think he looks around
and finds this world a funny place to live and
sometimes he laughs out loud. You can tell he sees things
are quite different, but they're not scary."

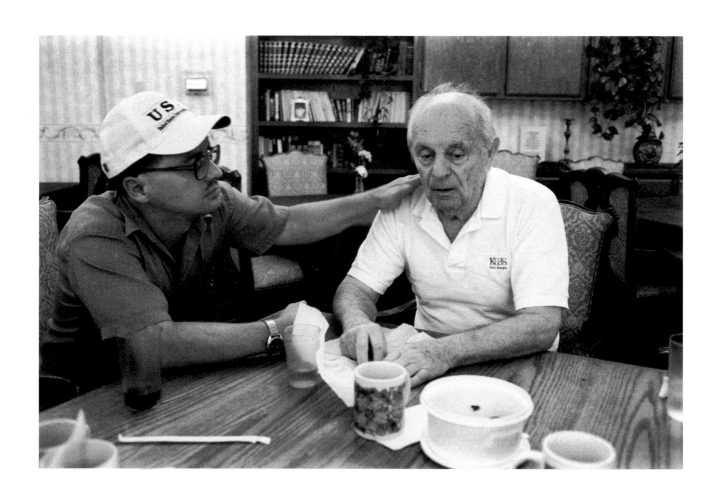

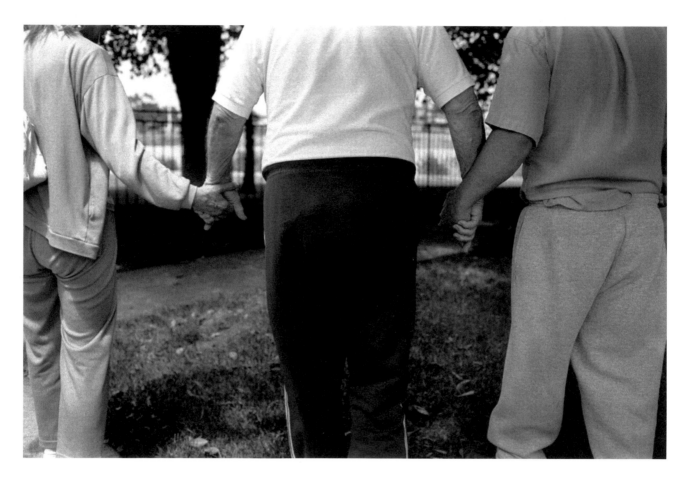

Igor and his family took long walks through the Silverado gardens.

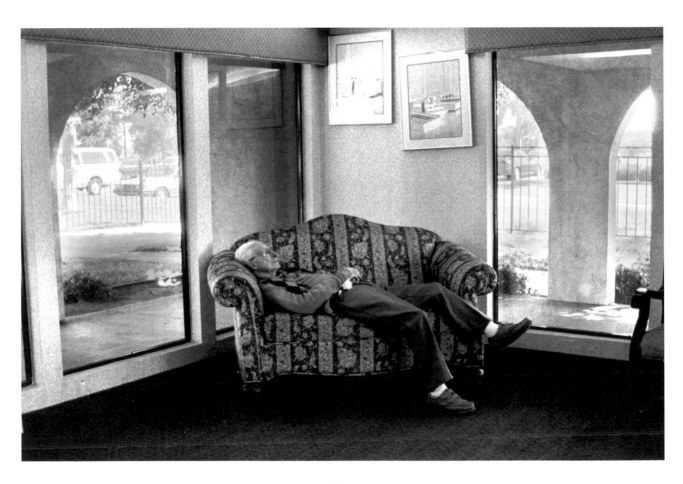

Silverado residents have freedom to move about the facility, inside and outside,
and to participate in activities or to "do their own thing."

Art was described to me as a gentle, caring, soft-spoken, diplomatic gentleman.
I met him only once, the day I joined six of the men on a Fourth of July outing to a nearby pool hall.
Art had a good time, although he didn't play pool. The next day I saw him napping in the main salon,
and he looked wonderfully peaceful. He died two days later.

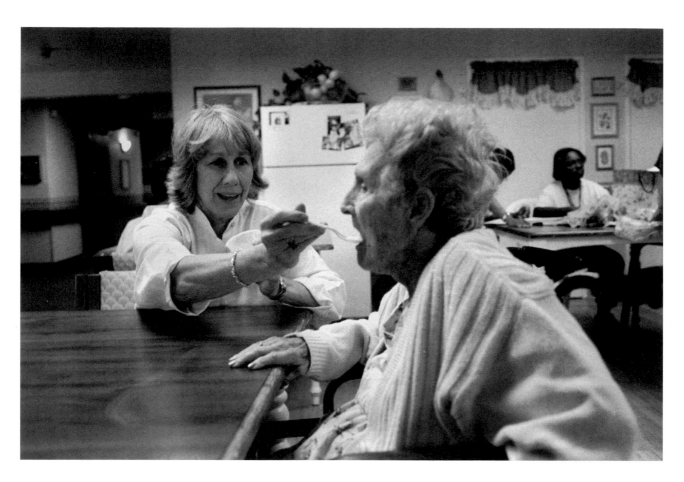

One Saturday Carole tried to feed MaryLou some ice cream. After I had photographed them a few times,
Carole said, "I'm so happy you're doing this. I know these will be the last photographs we will have of my mother.
She hasn't eaten for three days, and I know this is the end."

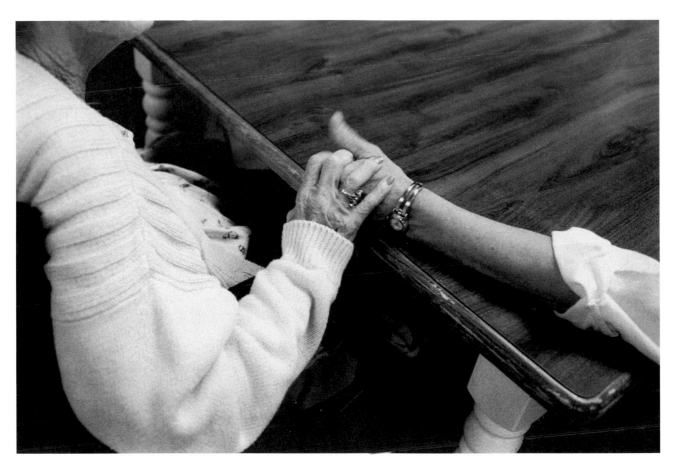

꧁

Later a caregiver told me she felt that MaryLou had lost her will to live. "They played bingo together, but they knew. MaryLou walked with her family that day, and she smiled a couple of times, but you could see in her face that she's had enough and she's tired. Her daughter cried. She didn't know what to do and how to do it. It was a difficult time, a painful time."

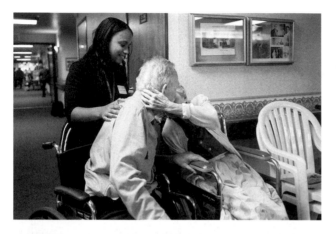
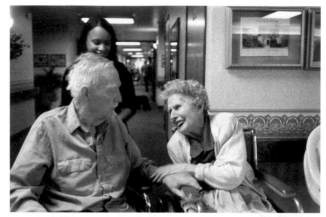
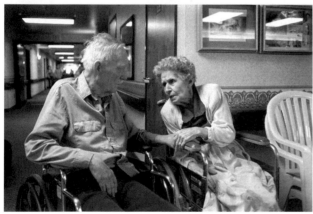
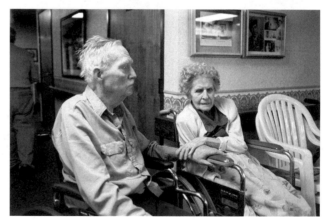

Clayton and Minna have been married for sixty years. Their daughter describes their marriage as a wonderful, happy one.
Minna has suffered from multiple sclerosis for the past forty years. It was difficult for her to make the decision three years ago that
Clayton could best be cared for at Silverado because of the advanced stage of his Alzheimer's. Soon thereafter,
Minna's Alzheimer's had advanced enough that she, too, moved to Silverado.

Clayton's illness had already reached a late stage when I was at Silverado. He and Minna lived in different rooms,
but when his condition permitted, Larissa or another caregiver would bring him out to the salon. Minna was always happy to see him.
They shared moments of tenderness and love for each other despite their serious health problems.

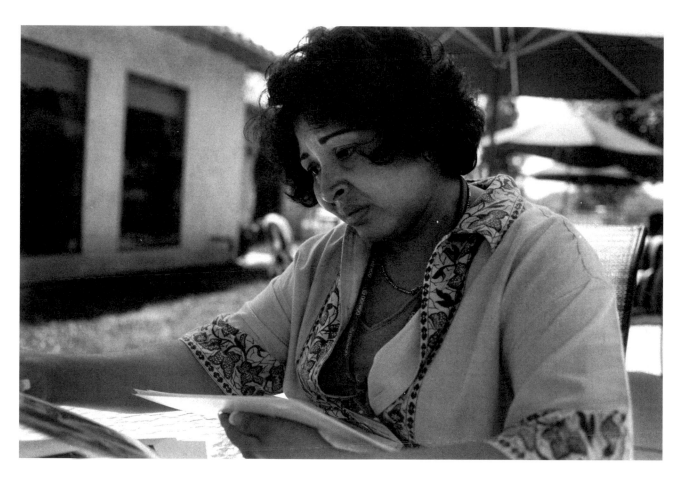

Miriam enjoyed looking at my photographs and talking about her work as a caregiver.
When she came to an image of a resident who had died the week before, her face changed completely.

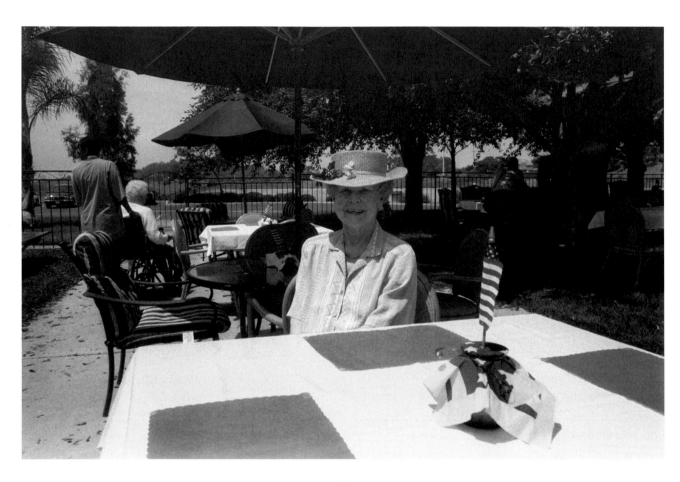

❦

"Meredith's husband comes here every morning. Jim arrives at her door and he'll spook her or scare her! And she just laughs, and they go hand in hand for a walk, and then they go to breakfast. It's a wonderful family, a close-knit family. The children have all been professionally successful, and when they come to visit they all sing together."

—a caregiver

Meredith liked to look elegant and a little sporty every day.
She was one of the first to be seated in the garden for the Fourth of July party.

A friend is someone who knows
the song in your heart
and can sing it back to you
when you have forgotten
the words.

Unknown

3

Filling the Silent Spaces

WHY DID I FIND SILVERADO TO BE SO SPECIAL? There were several reasons.

In many institutional settings, dementia patients are treated as frail, elderly patients to be managed. This approach compounds their disconnection. It soon becomes difficult to find any spirit in the body, much less the person who used to be there. In *Life Worth Living*, Dr. William Thomas writes: "Current practice in long-term care is based on a confusion of care, treatment, and kindness. Lying at the root of this confusion is the medical model's fixation on diagnosis and treatment. It guarantees that the majority of our resources are spent on the war against disease, when, in fact, loneliness, helplessness, and boredom steadily decay our nursing home residents' spirit" (p. 1).

A major problem today is that nursing home patients are overtreated everywhere: they are prescribed more than six different daily medications on average, often at a cost of $200–$400 per month. Thomas points out that "more than half the 1.7 million nursing home residents in the U.S. receive regular doses of psychotropic medications, which are particularly dangerous for the frail elderly" (p. 19). This, he argues, means that "it is often difficult to distinguish what is due to disease and what is caused by the treatment of disease" (p. 47).

The care practices at Silverado demonstrate that the Alzheimer's sufferers' connections to others and to their own past lives can be sustained at a far higher level than is generally believed. Each day I gathered more evidence of how "alive" these residents were compared to all other Alzheimer's sufferers I had seen. I tried to understand the sources of this higher level of functioning. It was not that they were less ill; indeed, these patients were all in the middle and later stages of the disease.

I became convinced that there were five critical sources of the extraordinary intensity I witnessed:

- a philosophy of care that emphasizes quality of life, achieved through careful monitoring, social stimulation, dietary regulation, and a supportive environment that stresses life purpose;

- a substantial reduction in the use of psychotropic medications, including antipsychotics, antianxieties, hypnotics, and antidepressants, among Silverado residents (though antidepressants are still an important part of their care);
- a staff well trained in dementia care and rewarded for respecting and honoring the "personhood" of each resident;
- the power of touch and physical contact; and
- the power of music, both in general use and in the specialized work of a certified music therapist.

"Easing your burden by creating a positive, fulfilling life for your loved one in a warm, comfortable, and compassionate setting": these are not just words in the literature sent to people considering a placement. This goal is part of the daily routine at Silverado. Personalized care plans build on residents' strengths, enhance positive self-image, and promote autonomy. This was clearly expressed when Pat, the program director, talked to me about her work:

> Whenever you do something that I call respecting their minds and letting them decide what they would like to have and do, it always works best. It is too easy to tell them what to do or to do it for them. But we are not working with brain dead people, we're working with brain damaged people. They're not incapable of learning, so we need always to be pushing, with very soft hands, but pushing to the maximum of their abilities and what they are able to do.
>
> They should be absolutely given choices. From the time they get up in the morning until they go to bed, they should be given choices. That's what the whole environment is about. It says, "You have a choice: a choice to live here in an open environment; to go inside

or out; to eat whenever you want to; to have visitors anytime you want, day or night; to go to the refrigerator when you want; to make your own coffee or tea or have your cookies with it; to have your own animal with you, whether it be a bird, a dog, a fish, or a rabbit. This environment sets the stage to say, *You* decide." When we don't cue them to it, we're not taking advantage of all the things that have been done; we're not really using the stage, so to speak.

The staff is the key to making this work. In addition to the director and the administrative staff, the expert team includes a registered nurse and a master's-level social worker—activity and research professionals who work together at all times. Consulting physicians visit frequently.

As is the practice in nursing homes and assisted living facilities, the certified nursing assistants who work in each wing are called *caregivers*. These people, including the receptionist at the front desk, are all trained in specialized dementia care. These front-line caregivers regularly receive information about the needs and preferences of the residents (who are never referred to as *patients*).

At the first staff meeting I attended, results of a competition to see who knew the most about the backgrounds of the residents were announced. Almost all the caregivers had high scores on the quiz, which included such questions as: Who played golf until she was eighty and was a fabulous gourmet cook? Who was a registered nurse in the military? Who was an engineer and built dams along the Rio Grande? and Who was born in Minnesota and loves to listen to baseball?

Careful recruiting, ongoing training, high wages, regular staff meetings, staff empowerment, and constant reinforcement of the importance of creating relationships with the residents keep the staff turnover rate far below the industry-wide average. They also result in high levels of satisfaction among residents and family members, including Renee, the daughter of a former resident: "I delayed placement for my mother for fear that she would not receive the love and respect that she deserved. How wrong I was! During her life at Silverado, she was showered with affection, stimulated by the joyous atmosphere of loving pets and darling children, and indeed, treated with honor and dignity. In addition to all this, they welcomed my participation in her care and made me feel part of the Silverado family. I will forever be thankful for the opportunity to stay with her during her final days, allowing us to be together until the end. She died in peace and comfort, surrounded by love."

The importance of a hug, a caress of the cheek, the holding of hands is seldom forgotten at Silverado. Caregivers as well as family visitors embrace and give loving touches to the residents. Staff members' children are frequently present and provide physical contact as well as visual stimulation for the residents. Many tensions are reduced by just a few moments spent petting one of the dogs or cats living at the facility. The power of touch is evident in its frequent results: moments of connection and sometimes joy, a softened facial expression, a smile, the making and holding of eye contact.

After my field work at Silverado, I found documents about the power of touch as a key element of care. Marie de Hennezel's writings on life and death contain repeated references to her own training in haptonomy, the science of affective contact, training she asks the rest of her staff at a hospital for palliative care in Paris to take as well. Recounting her experience with one dying patient, Louis, de Hennezel says the following, which captures much of what I felt at Silverado: "He seems to need gentle, silent contact. He likes it when I softly lay my hands on his sick eyes and on all the places on his body that hurt him—his legs, his clenched solar plexus. He likes the feeling of being touched with physical respect: it makes him feel he's still a living human being. He once described this kind of attention that my hands are giving him as 'caressing the soul.' . . . Sometimes there is no substitute for the touch of a hand" (de Hennezel 1998, p. 158).

Liberty, choices, the regular presence of children and pets, a rich program of optional activities including outings, caregiving with respect and love, physical contact—each greatly impressed me for its powerful impact on the residents. But I was unprepared for the important role music can play. There were many other art programs and activities, but none impressed me the way music did. Chapters 4 and 5 address what I felt was the "magic" of music in keeping people who are living with Alzheimer's disease truly alive.

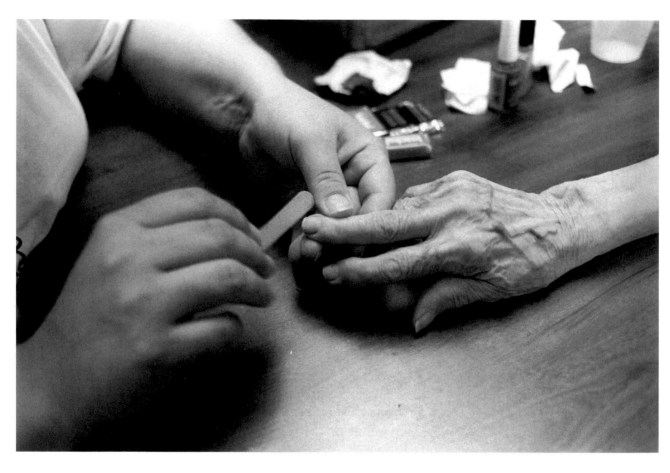

The staff at Silverado foster positive self-image by helping the residents be well dressed and well groomed.
Something as simple as having a manicure can also be a source of much pleasure.
Hilda was happy to receive the attention from one of the caregivers, and she was happy that her hands looked good afterward.

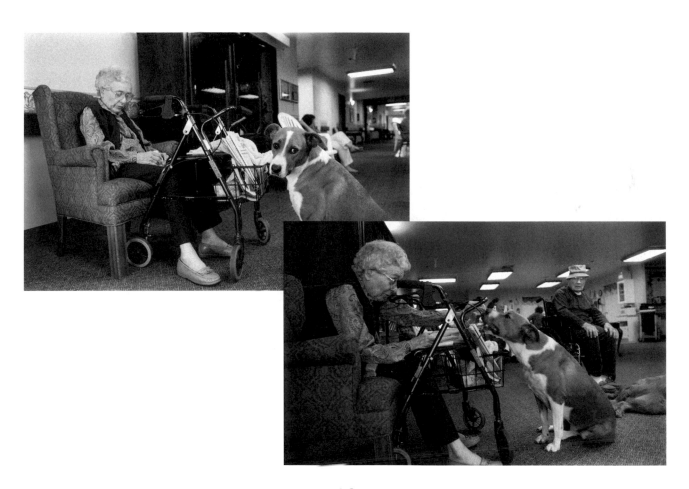

⌘

"One of the things I love about this place is how they make it so homelike with the pets. They're so wonderful!
I've seen a lot of residents who aren't very responsive to anything, but if a dog or a cat walks up, they're immediately there,
they're present, they're reaching down to pet them."
—a family member

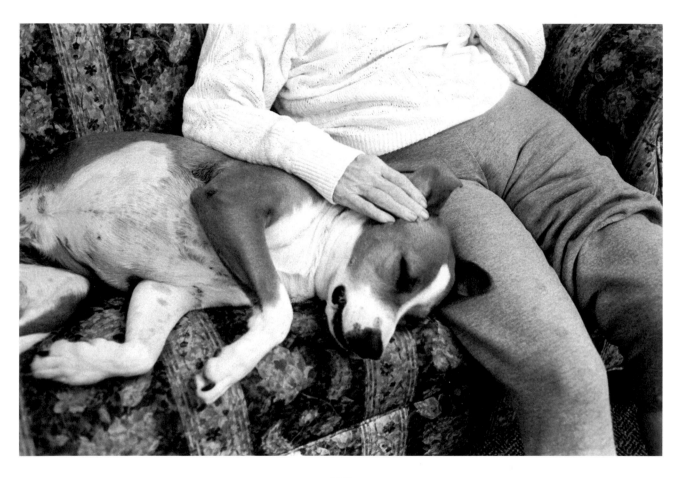

❧

"I think these furry animals bring a lot of life into these people. They're always reaching, and if they don't have someone, they've got that little dog or cat, and there's a chance to show love. And who knows, maybe it brings back a memory of something warm, like sitting in front of a fireplace with their family, or their old dog if they had one. But whatever their thoughts are, the contact creates a relaxation and a sense of connection."

—Sue, a caregiver

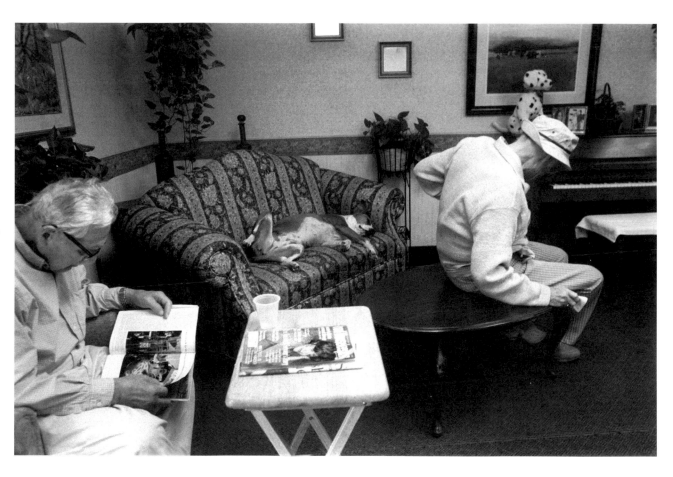

Some residents bring their pets with them when they move to Silverado. These animals often remain at the facility after their owners' deaths. Others, like Abby, were acquired by the staff.

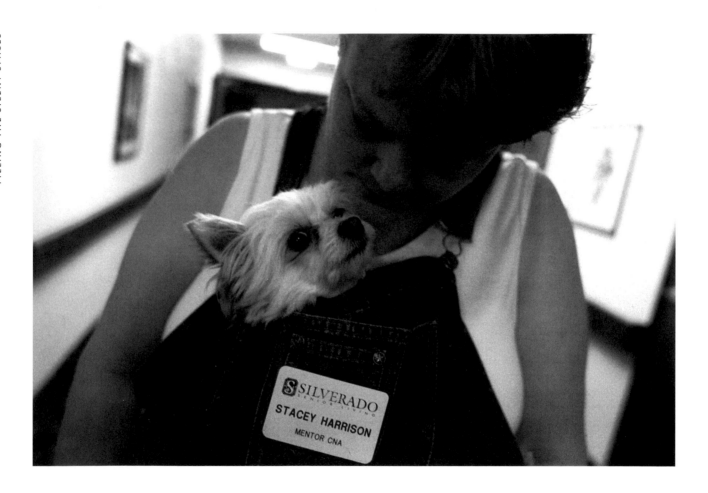

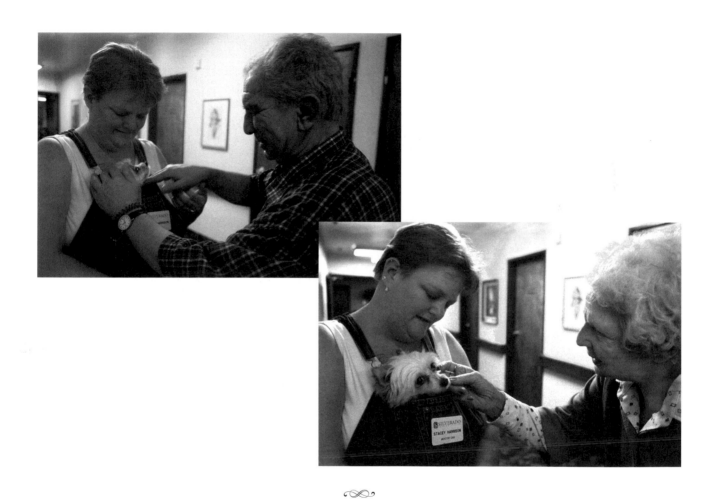

Dorothy smiles often, and Phil smiles occasionally. Both were captivated when Stacey brought her dog, Roxy, to work.

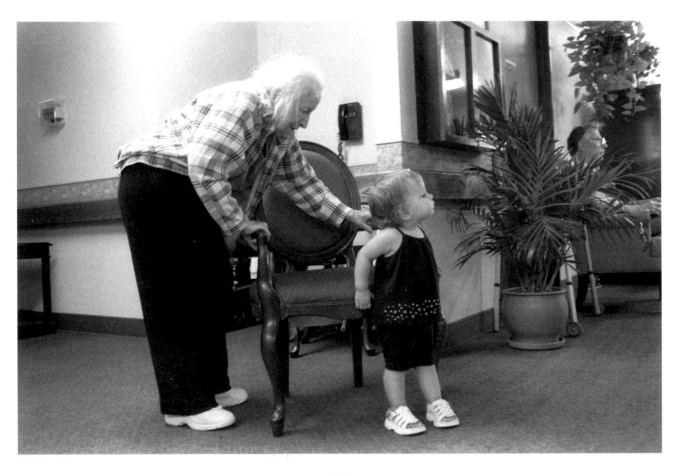

The presence of children always brings a smile, a laugh, or a caress. Often the residents, even those who are usually silent, will initiate conversations.

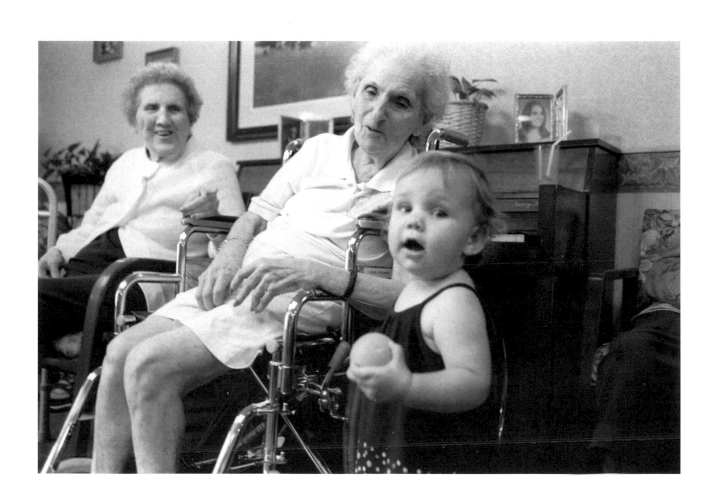

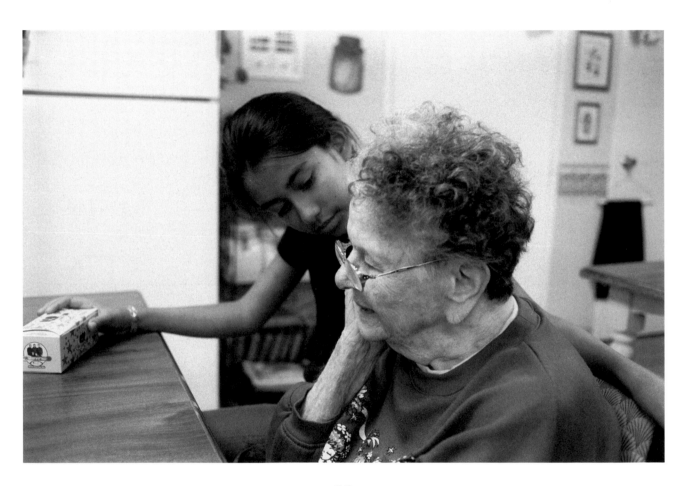

Melissa, the daughter of one of the caregivers, was sweet to everyone and completely at ease with the residents.
It didn't seem to matter to her that they often didn't communicate clearly in words.

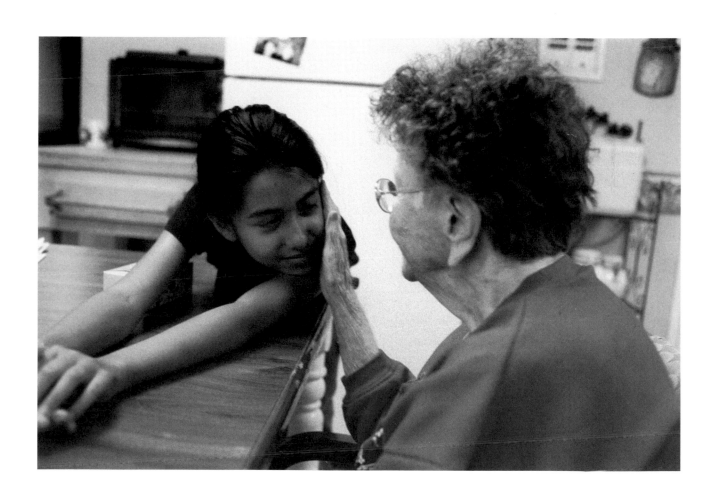

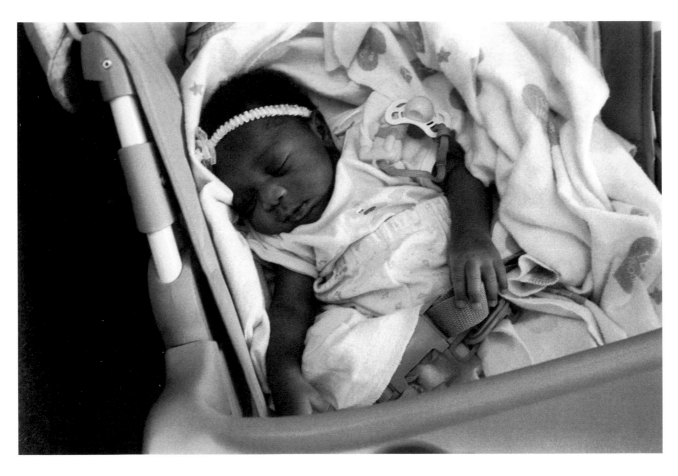

The youngest "visitor" I saw at Silverado was the newborn child of one of the staff members.
Her mother was on maternity leave but had returned for a baby shower and "parade" through
both wings when the infant was a week old.

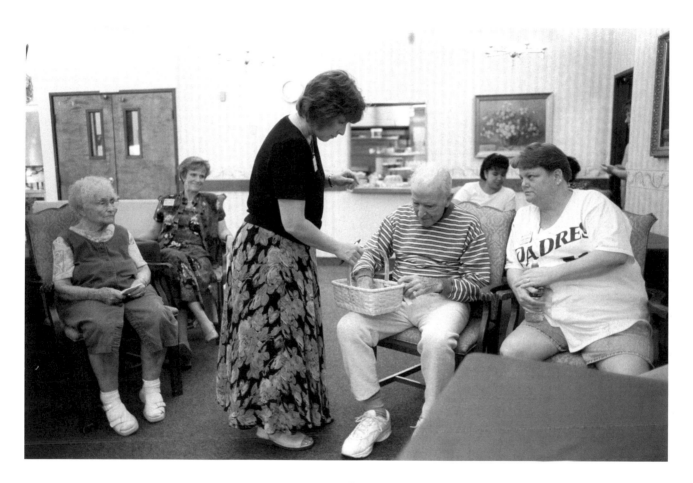

When Tom and Elsie wandered into a staff meeting, no one batted an eye. Kathy Greene, the director,
asked Tom to help by picking a name from a basket. Elsie was a nurse when she was younger;
in confused moments she thinks she is one of the Silverado staff members. During the meeting, she announced,
"I quit!! I'm 87 and too old to work these ten-hour shifts you give me!" Kathy treated the statement seriously
and promised to cut Elsie's hours. She also took the opportunity to tell Elsie, "You are invaluable."

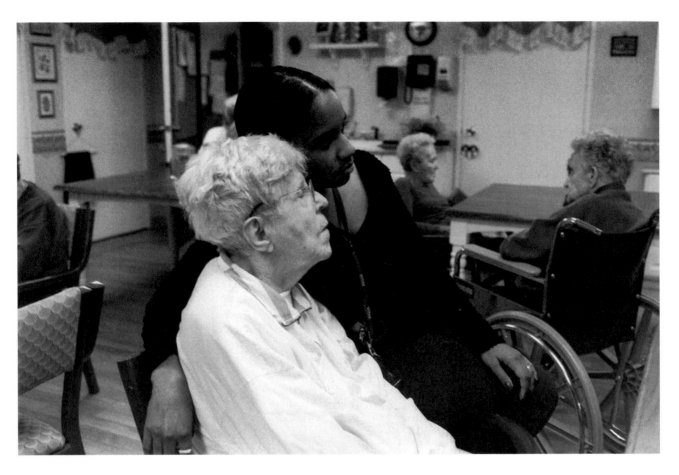

Quality caregiving includes spending quiet time with residents when they need companionship and loving,
which Larissa frequently offered to those in her wing.

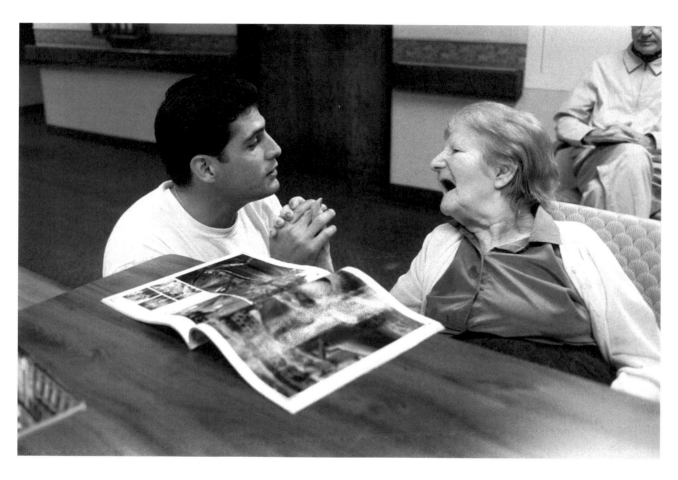

Like some of the other residents, Carmella loved it when Kevin, a caregiver, called her Grandma.

Dr. Rockwell, looking at this photograph, commented, "You can get so carried away with these wonderful people and their need. I think that's what pulled me into geriatrics. . . . Suddenly you're working with people who appreciate you and just drink you up, and it is a wonderful feeling. There are so many people reaching out, trying to grab your hand, and you leave feeling guilty for what you can't give them."

7
8:30AM	MUSIC THERAPY (WEST WING)
9:30A	NEWS/COFFEE
10AM	EXERCISE
11AM	EMBLEM BELLS
11AM	LIFE ENHANCEMENT
1:15P	BAKE SHOPPE
2PM	TABLE GAMES
5:15PM	STORY TIME
7PM	SMALL GROUP ACTIVITIES

8
9:30A	NEWS/COFFEE
10AM	OUTING
11AM	EXERCISE
1:15P	BAKE SHOPPE
2:15P	BINGO
3PM	WANDERLUST
5:15P	STORY TIME
3:15PM	LIFE STORIES
7PM	SMALL GROUP ACTIVITIES

9
8:45A	CATHOLIC MASS
9:00AM	ARTS & CRAFTS W/LINDA
10AM	NEWS/COFFEE
11AM	EXERCISE
2PM	SPECIAL ENTERTAINMENT W/JOHNNY LONG
3:30P	UNO
5:15P	STORY TIME
7PM	SMALL GROUP ACTIVITIES

10
8:30AM	MUSIC THERA...
9:00AM	COOKING C...
1:15PM	BAKE SHO...
2PM	TEA PAR...
3PM	MOVIE/P...
5:15P	STORY T...
7PM	SMALL G...

14
	MUSIC THERAPY (WEST WING)
	NEWS/COFFEE
	EXERCISE
	LIFE ENHANCEMENT
	BAKE SHOPPE
	TABLE GAMES
	STORY TIME
	SMALL GROUP ACTIVITIES

15 — *MEN'S CLUB TO HORSE RACES*
9:30A	NEWS/COFFEE
10AM	OUTING
11AM	EXERCISE
1:15P	BAKE SHOPPE
2:15P	BINGO
3PM	WANDERLUST
3:15PM	LIFE STORIES
5:15P	STORY TIME
7PM	SMALL GROUP ACTIVITIES

16
8:45A	CATHOLIC MASS
9:00AM	ARTS & CRAFTS W/LINDA
10AM	NEWS/COFFEE
11AM	EXERCISE
2PM	SPECIAL ENTERTAINMENT W/BRUCE RADDER
3:30P	UNO
5:15P	STORY TIME
7PM	SMALL GROUP ACTIVITIES

17
8:30AM	MUSIC...
9:00AM	COO...
1:15PM	BAK...
2PM	TEA...
3PM	MO...
5:15P	ST...
7PM	SM...

(21)
	MUSIC THERAPY (WEST WING)
	NEWS/COFFEE
	EXERCISE
	LIFE ENHANCEMENT
	BAKE SHOPPE
	TABLE GAMES
	STORY TIME
	SMALL GROUP ACTIVITIES

22
9:30A	NEWS/COFFEE
10AM	OUTING
11AM	EXERCISE
1:15P	BAKE SHOPPE
12NOON	HAWAIIAN LUAU
2:15P	BINGO
3PM	WANDERLUST
3:15PM	LIFE STORIES
5:15P	STORY TIME
7PM	SMALL GROUP ACTIVITIES

23
8:45A	CATHOLIC MASS
9:00AM	ARTS & CRAFTS W/LINDA
10AM	NEWS/COFFEE
11AM	EXERCISE
2PM	SPECIAL ENTERTAINMENT W/JOHN MORAN
3:30P	UNO
5:15P	STORY TIME
7PM	SMALL GROUP ACTIVITIES

24
8:30AM	
9:00AM	
1:15PM	
2PM	
3PM	
5:15P	
7PM	

Most residents found several activities they could enjoy on the busy schedule of events.

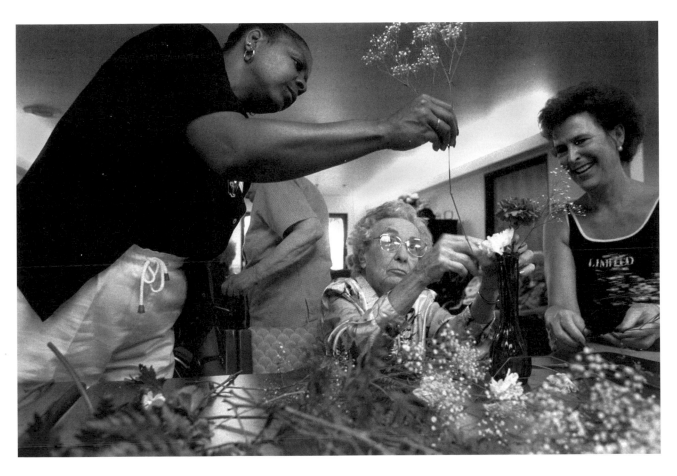

"Mrs. O'Leary is so determined to make everything right, whether it's a bouquet of flowers or anything. That's the way she's lived her life—she has been quite a lady. Something like this is difficult for her now, but she always does her best. She's becoming bonded, starting to feel that this is her home. At one time she thought of dying because this just was not her real home, but recently she's picked up, and she enjoys doing things now. She reaches out, pets the little dogs, and gets a kick out of things. And Barbara, a wonderful English lady from her neighborhood, comes all the time, and her visits just brighten up Mrs. O'Leary's day."

—Sue, a caregiver

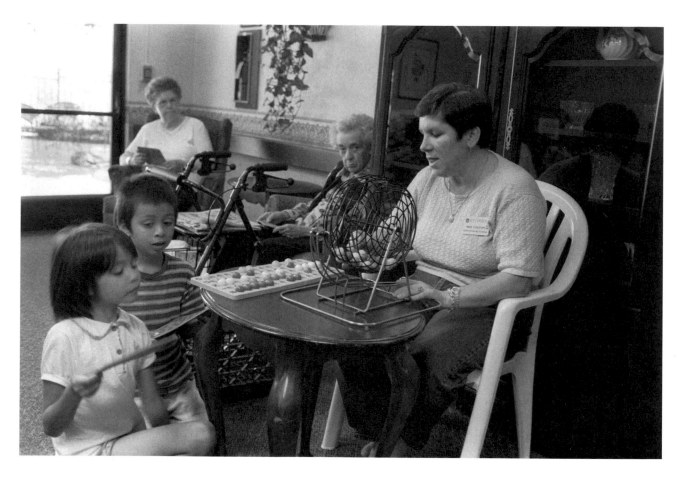

Iman ran a bingo game a few times a week. Anyone who wanted to play joined in the game, using small boards with sliders so there were no chips to drop.

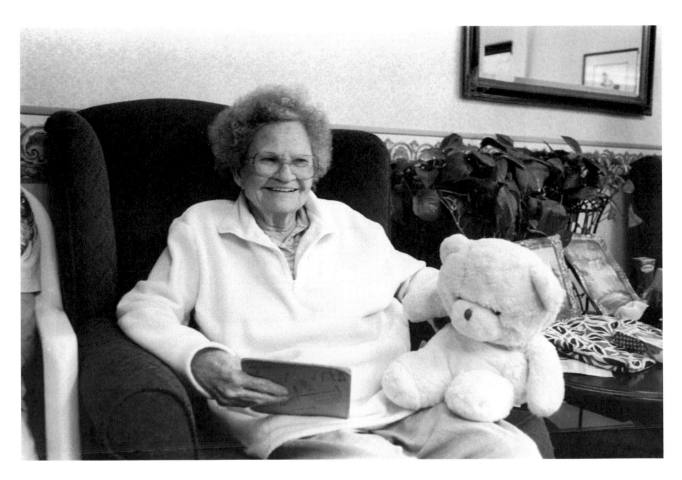

Sadie Mae won four of the six bingo games this day. She delighted in the attention and the astonishment that her extraordinary run of luck generated. She was also pleased by her prizes.

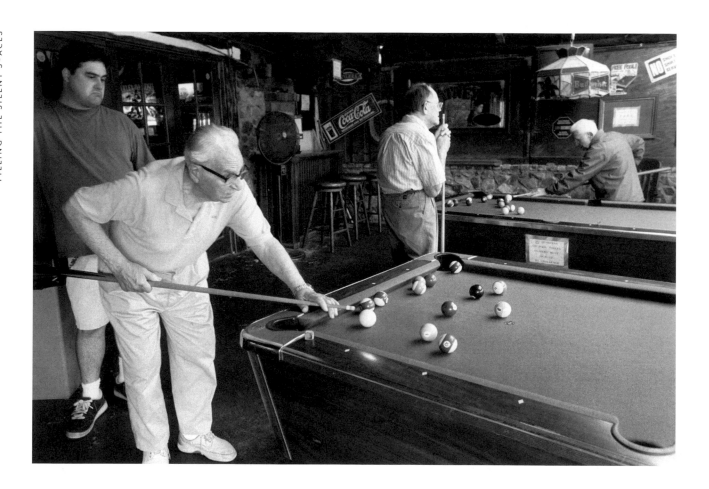

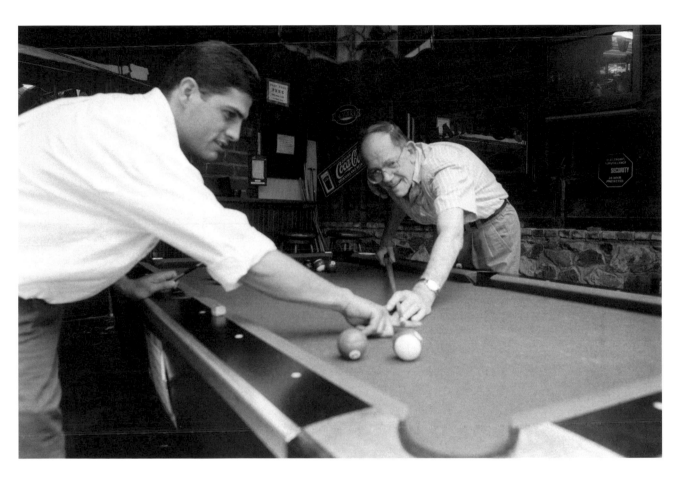

An excursion to a local pool hall was fun even for those who didn't remember all the rules. They found challenge and pleasure in just hitting the balls into the holes. And afterward there was cold beer, big hamburgers, and fries. The next week, Dan and Kevin organized a trip to a Padres baseball game, and the week after, Iman brought ten residents to her home for a barbecue.

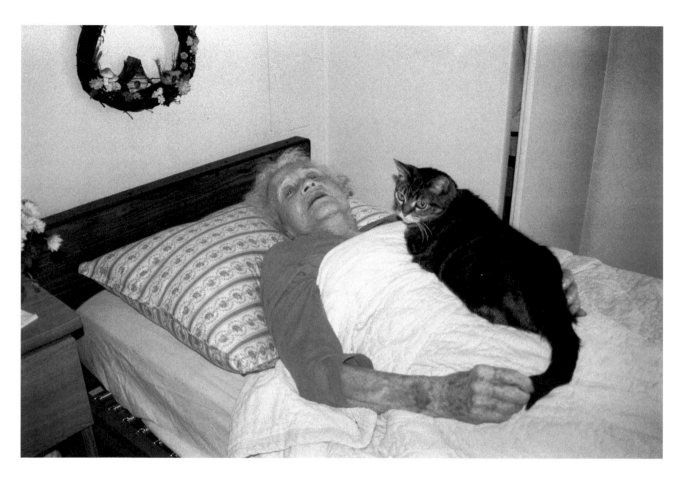

Edith had recently moved from another institution, where she had been heavily medicated for two years.
In her early days at Silverado she was often bedridden, and she enjoyed Cricket's companionship.

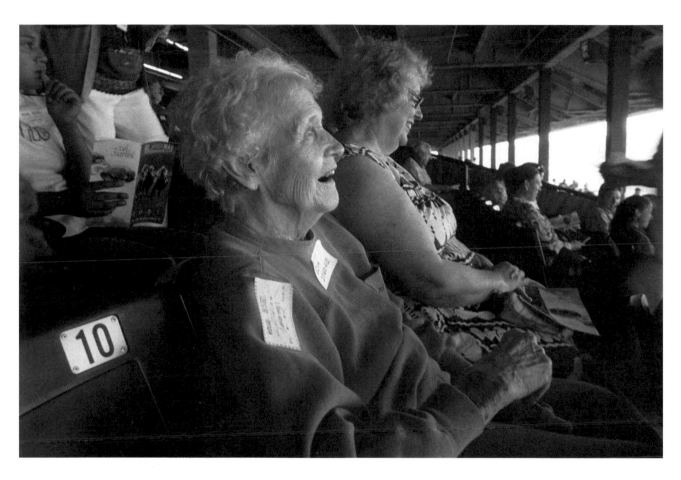

A month later Edith joined a group of residents and her daughter on an excursion to the Del Mar racetrack.
It was hard to believe that she had been bedridden until only a few weeks earlier.

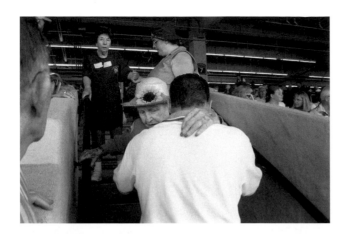
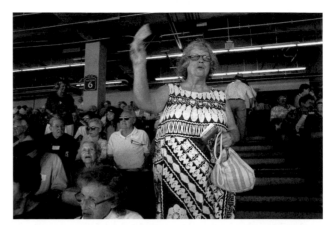
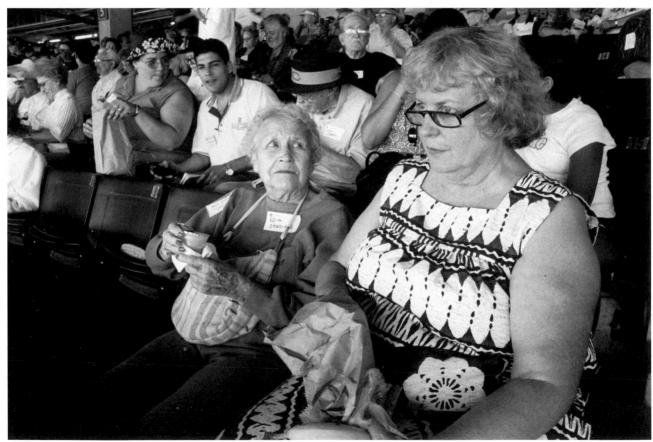

An Excursion to the Racetrack

CATHY GREENBLAT: Kevin, I had such a wonderful time the other day on the excursion to the racetrack. You must have been both exhausted and exhilarated when you got back. I'd love to hear how you feel about it now.

KEVIN (A CAREGIVER): What I wanted to do was to take some of the residents who I thought would enjoy the races on an excursion to the Del Mar track. We have a lot of people here from substantial backgrounds, and many of them used to go to the track when they were healthy. . . . It's all about quality of life—that's one of our mottoes here—and I felt that some of our residents would really like it. It was not so much for the betting but for the horses, but some liked the betting, while some just liked the event itself, being out in the public.

CATHY: Did you know in advance who would be going?

KEVIN: The whole thing was on a balance until that day. We had people on the list to go, but we always have to see at the last minute, because certain people have their peaks and valleys, they either perform very well or they don't perform very well at all. We had to see that day how each one was. We have to weigh all aspects of the person to decide whether they can go, because there have been incidents where we've taken someone out, and they've formed their own sense of independence all of a sudden and said, "I'm not going back with you, my house is just around the corner." We know they have the ability to be combative to a degree, and we sometimes chance it.

They loved it. There was one person in particular I think of, Larry. He's a big cat-napper—he'll sleep on and off the whole day—but the entire time he was there his attention was focused on what was going on around him or on the races themselves. That was a plus for us. Then the reaction I got from his wife when I came back and told her about the day, that was a reward in itself, because she's seeing the deterioration of the man that she knew. So learning that he had a good time and that it brought something out in him made her cry, and then it got to us, too, and we cried.

One of the other people I think about is Sadie Mae. She really enjoyed the bets; she was having a good time watching the horses. She got a little restless toward the end, but she likes to get out and do that kind of thing.

And the palling around was more with John and Howard. They kind of stuck to me, you know: "Where's Kevin?" As long as they saw me there, it was OK. And Howard, we had a couple of great moments, like when we saw the big-chested woman walk by. We both were looking down, and as we looked up at the same time and caught each other's eye, and it was just like a special moment in time. This woman walked by, and she was gorgeous, and we stared at her chest and then looked at each other, and we both sort of blushed, like "Holy Moses!" and he was saying, "Holy Toledo, ay chi mama!" And we just couldn't stop laughing.

The other incident with Howard was when we had to go to the restroom. I had them all lined up at the urinals, and Howard was in between two people who were not in our group. There was an older man and a younger gentleman. So he was at the urinal, and suddenly he said, "Gosh that water's cold! And deep, too!" And I got the joke and started laughing. The older gentleman leaned back kind of to see "How big are you?!" It was funny!

And then of course there's Edith. I think she and her daughter had the best time of everyone, because of the mother-daughter thing. Edith liked the horses; the daughter liked the betting. She loved seeing her mother there, enjoying herself.

CATHY: You parked the van, and somebody took

Edith and Larry over in their wheelchairs, because they were the first ones there . . .

KEVIN: Yes, everybody at the track was really great. We had a group rate, but they weren't aware of what kind of a group of people we were bringing. But when they saw, they were very quick to react. We had a little minivan come that was wheelchair accessible, and the driver said he would take anyone over that needed it. So Mr. James was one and Edith was another who arrived from the parking lot in that minivan. Edith could walk at that point, but we didn't want to tire her out because as you know we had some steps she had to walk later.

CATHY: As you remember, I arrived there before the bus came. I had been talking to an employee who was steering people to the correct entry gate. I told her I was waiting for "my group" and that they were elderly people with Alzheimer's. Later she pointed out a woman with her back to us, next to a man in a wheelchair, who also had his back to us. He was sitting with his body slumped to one side. The employee said to me, "How can he enjoy the track?" Not knowing who the man was, I said, "The problem is that we look at him and ask how he can enjoy it compared to you or me, who are in better health. But maybe that's the wrong question. . . . Maybe we have to ask how he can enjoy the track compared to whatever else he would be doing if he were not here."

KEVIN: Exactly.

CATHY: And she said, "Oh that's interesting! I hadn't thought about it that way." A minute later you arrived, and Edith's daughter and Larry turned around, and I realized they were part of our group. Then we went inside, and there was the place to park the wheelchairs, but Larry didn't want to be there and you helped him to a seat . . .

KEVIN: He decided. You know his whole view is restricted because when he sees things, he sees his knees and his feet. Because of his disease, he's got that posture and it's really hard for him to keep his head up. But I explained what was going on, and I held his chin up and said, "That's what's going on over there, and we're going to place our bets over there . . ." I asked him if he had ever been here, and he said, "Yes, it's been some time, but we used to come every now and then." He started to get a little restless, and I said, "Do you need something?" and he said, "Yes, I feel I should be down below with the rest of the group, not here in the wheelchair section." That's how I knew he was very interested in what was going on. It was his choice. And even with the stairs and all, the obstacle of getting down there, he wanted to sit with the rest of us, and that was just great. So I helped him and I helped Edith get to the seats.

I got him last after everyone else was seated, and he had been sitting up there so long his legs were rubber from inactivity. Our group was sitting about midway down the stairs, and I started to lift Larry, but it took a little time to get his legs to offer enough stability. Then a gentleman popped up and said, "Can I help you?" I said, "That would be great." While he helped, he said, "I totally feel great about what you guys are doing because my father recently passed away, and I totally appreciate what you're doing." And I thanked him, and Larry looked up and said, "Thank you," just as clear as could be.

There were a couple of other assisted living communities that had groups there, not the residents themselves, but the staff, and several of them said, "We have Alzheimer's units, and we're amazed at what you are doing with these people."

CATHY: I don't think many residents on dementia units have such opportunities.

KEVIN: I don't know if you noticed, but we got a fifty-fifty reaction while we were there . . . from other people. It was either they were very appreciative or we were treated like we were bothersome. Remember when you said, "We're with a group," and that lady said, "Well, I'm with a group, too," and she pushed her way in through the entry? She was very adamant about going through. I understand they are there to have a good time, but they feel like our people are inappropriate, they are in their way, they remind them of things they don't want to think about when they're out having a good time.

Remember we had that group that came in, that family, and they insisted that we move so they could take their exact seats? We had that back row completely open and they could have sat back there, but those were the tickets they had, and he wanted those seats. He would rather disrupt the whole thing and move everybody for his own satisfaction. And others now and then showed that they felt "we're here to make our bets, and you're in our way."

It's unfortunate, but that's what some of our society's views are about what this disease is, and some people feel we should keep them hidden away. I just pray this disease never happens to those families because they're going to have to learn to deal with this.

And then the other half, like the gentleman who helped me, or the woman who took the bets, or the guy who helped us with the wheelchair, thought it was fantastic that we were taking them out, bringing them here. Some people sitting around us were helping to keep an eye on them and said, "That's really great."

Did you see the slight anxiousness in the last hour? It started off with one person. That's kind of how our place is, and what dealing with these people is like. It starts off as a spark, and all of a sudden you have a fire going. . . . It goes from one energy to the next. You start to see the whole thing moving around.

CATHY: It was all under control, but I was hearing it from a lot of places. . . . In the last hour I couldn't photograph because Maureen had grabbed one of my hands and was hanging on tightly, and Daphne was clutching my other hand, so I had no hand for the camera!

KEVIN: In the bus back, there were different reactions. Howard had a good time, and he could kind of recollect. Larry had a good time, but he was much more into the view on the drive there and back. As I said, he spends so much of the time looking down, and now he was holding his head up because he really wanted to see.

As we were going through the mountains of Rancho Santa Fe, Al was pointing out some of the areas he used to work in. Sadie Mae was worried and kept asking, "Are we going to miss dinner?" John was a little anxious because we were back on a bus and he thought he was going home, and he was concerned about not remembering where he had parked his car. And Daphne just wanted to be sure I was there. She felt that I was her strong connection. We caught a little traffic, they got a little restless on the bus, but they did well. Everybody did well. I was ready to fall apart!

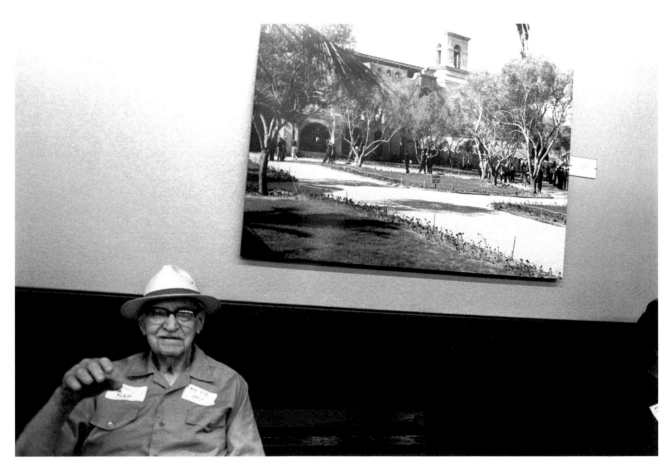

Abe was happier than I had ever seen him when he took a rest under the big poster of the race track.
He asked me to take his photo there.

4

Bringing Back the Songs

I ADMIRED HILDA FOR HER LOVELY SPIRIT. It was Hilda who first introduced me to what ultimately impressed me greatly as a means for staying alive: music as a way of maintaining connections to the past and to other people.

Hilda had come to Silverado with her piano two years earlier. She played it occasionally, but more often she played the small upright piano in the lounge near her room. Each day she sat at the bench, waiting for someone to call out the name of a favorite song. Then she began to play each requested song. Every note was perfect, and she sang the words perfectly, too. Sometimes she played classical music. In those moments Hilda was not lost. And others in the room, many of whom were habitually quiet, began to sing along with words that came to them from their pasts.

Hilda frequently did not know whether she had eaten twenty minutes earlier. But at the piano she could recall and play and sing more than two hundred songs that made up her repertoire. Pat, the program director,

talked about Hilda and her music:

> Music was an essential part of her life and what makes her, it is her center. So no matter how much she is upset or having a bad day or just not happy with the world at the moment, we can make her happy, we can change her mood with music. . . . And because of her delight in it, she is able to delight others with it. And that is another thing, it is her communication skill now. She is not able to sit down and hold a full-fledged conversation with somebody or to initiate a conversation that makes totally good sense. She can say certain words, but a lot of it is word salad: she doesn't make a lot of sense most of the time. What she is able to do is to entertain with her music. With her music she can create a rapport with people and become recognized because of that. Everybody now sees Hilda and one of the first things that happens is that they think of her piano, they think of her music, just as you do when you see Hilda.

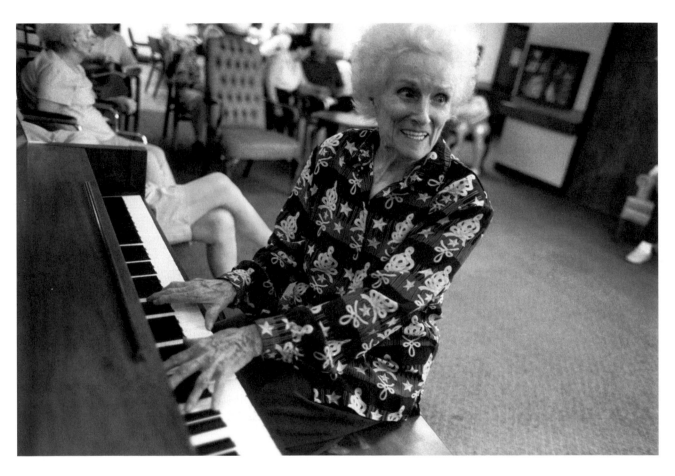

Once Hilda is given a title of a song she is able to go to her long-term memory and recall it.
Sometimes she can't do that, and you need to hum a melody, because she could not pull up the right information
with just the verbal cue. Once she hears the melody, it clicks in, and she's able to transfer
that information down to her fingers.

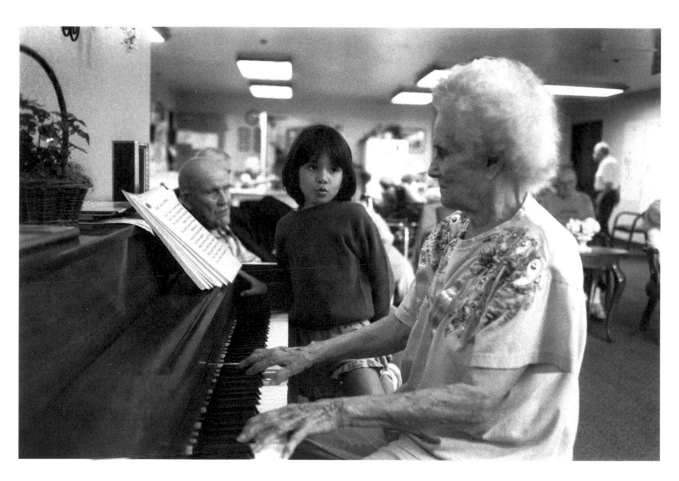

One Monday morning I saw a whiteboard placed near the piano in the east salon. Written on it was a list of songs:
"Somewhere over the Rainbow," "Home on the Range," "Danny Boy," "Oh Susanna."
In a large box was the phrase "Thank you, Hilda Larson. We love you."

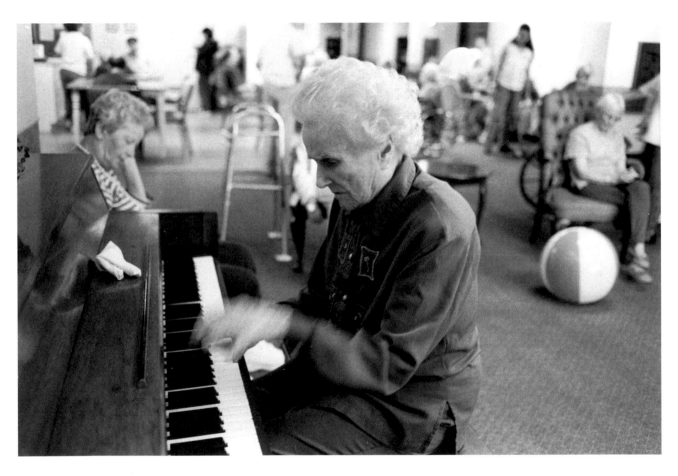

❧

"Hilda can play us a song that she learned forty, fifty, or even eighty years ago. And the sadness will come
if her disease progresses to a point that she can no longer transfer the information from her brain to
her fingers to make those keys jingle a little more. Those days for us will be sad; it will be sad to watch that happen."
—a caregiver

Pat had been a gospel singer for many years, and she still sang at her church. She developed the music program at Silverado. Pat has worked with dementia patients for two decades, and she believes strongly in the power of music.

I've never been formally taught about music. I'm a vocalist as you know. I have my own professional-size karaoke that I have here all the time with me. What makes music work for me here is that it's worked for me all my life. Being African American, a major part of my culture has been music and dancing. Number one, it was free. When we were poor, when we didn't have any money, we had to entertain each other. And music was our communication mode. We passed messages through it. As far back as you can go as an African American, everything happened with it.

Now I have two grandkids—I got my grandkids dancing even before they could walk. And I taught them songs, and they started singing them back as soon as they learned some words, and then they learned all the words. Dancing is so central, and singing brought us together, it made us one. When we come together as a family, with all our different interests, what unites us is music. I recognized how it brought us together, and it worked for everyone whether they were good at it or not

Pat often used music to change the tone of a group of residents in the public areas of the facility. If she felt a great deal of tension and anxiety among them, she played soft music. If the tone of the room was heavy or depressed, she played more energetic music. Often she used music to increase participation and interaction and connection. Watching her perform and seeing the transformation of the residents, I gained additional support for the idea that memories of music and its pleasures seem to survive long after other memories have dimmed or been lost.

Sometimes I just take out my karaoke system and start to sing. Within fifteen or twenty minutes you will see the residents who are habitually withdrawn come to sing with me, or begin to dance, or move their fingers or feet to the music, or just show a sign of recognition on their faces that they are connected. The music is what inspires dancing. . . .That's where my love and my passion comes from, it comes from my soul. And I like to think that's where my love for the residents comes from, so it makes sense that it all comes together and I'm able, with it, to draw them to me and to make us all a team. We have a fine time together.

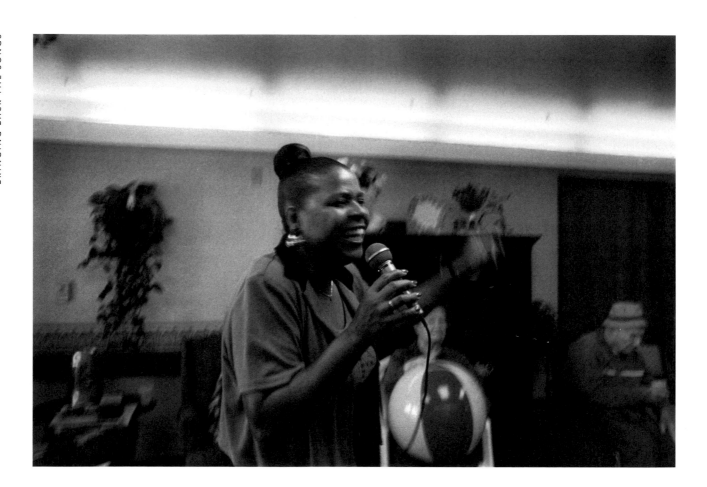

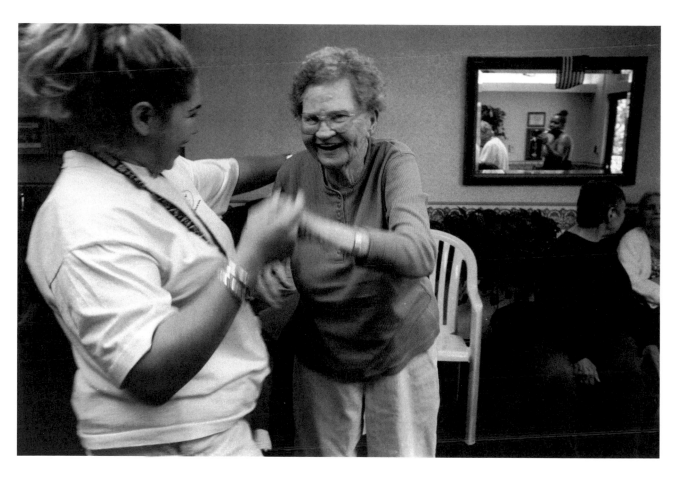

Dr. Rockwell, looking at these photos, exclaimed, "This is wonderful! These are the parts of the brain that are alive! You don't have to have a parietal lobe and a temporal lobe functioning at full steam to experience this kind of joy."

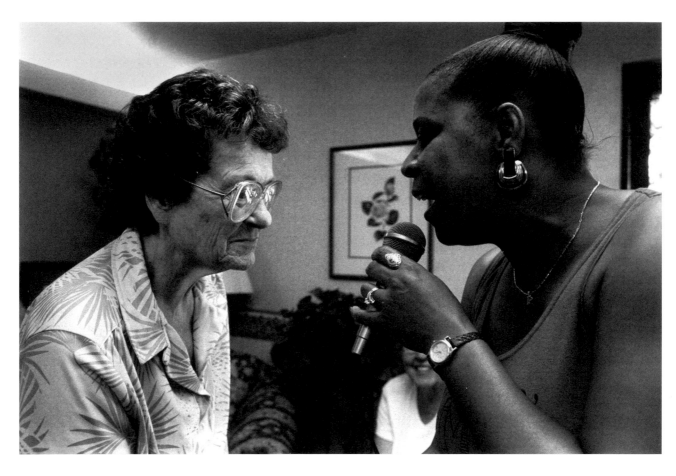

Liz was increasingly disconnected and withdrawn during the weeks I was at Silverado. But when Pat began singing,
Liz came right up to her and hummed along.

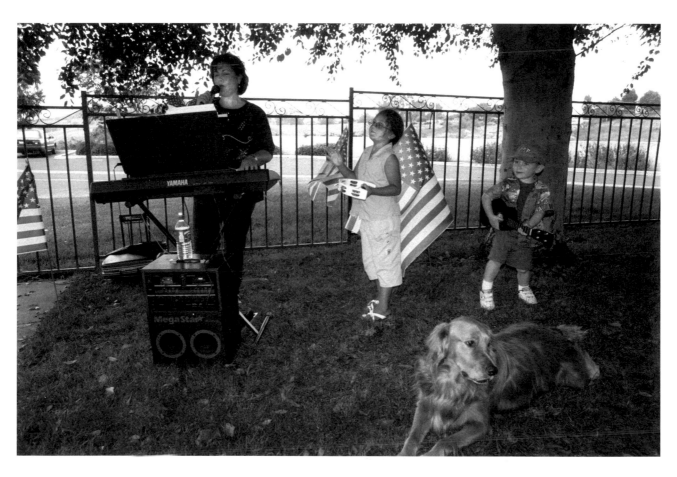

Music is central in the Silverado programming. There is special entertainment every Thursday and a paid entertainer one Saturday a month, one Friday a month, and two Sundays a month.

Everyone loved the sound of music at the Fourth of July party, offered by a paid entertainer, her son, and the daughter of one of the caregivers.

"Holding Hands without Touching"

Once again, Pat offered insight into why music is so effective in Alzheimer's care:

Working with dementia there are so many different activities that we offer but none of them work the way music does. If we are playing cards, everyone is out to win for themselves. If we're catching the ball, everyone is worried about how they catch the ball and not worried about the other guy. If we're playing board games or bingo, each one is hoping to win. Music is that one activity where we are all working with that one goal, to create one quality of sound, to stay on that same note. With music we are holding hands without touching. Its beauty is how we come together, synchronize and hold each other's hands.

Many of the residents who are usually quiet remember the words to songs when we start singing, because it is not threatening. The Alzheimer's victim is a master of deception. He has spent a lot of his time, many of his years, hiding his disability from people, and really he is embarrassed oftentimes at what he does not know. You know he recognizes his shortcomings, and he hates it that he has to show them all the time to people.

When we do an activity like music and they know that they know, it is easy to go ahead and start mouthing those words, and they are very comfortable. This is not a threatening activity. They can feel, "I don't have to be the loudest voice in the room" because whoever is leading the activity is normally the loudest voice in the room. Adding your voice to the chorus of the sound is not going to delete or add so much to it. They are not taking too many risks in singing the song, and they don't want to be called out when they forget a portion of the song. They make a comeback when they remember the portion that they know, and they can feel strong and good about it, but they didn't make or break the dynamics of what is going on.

So music is that one activity that brings us all together and keeps us standing as one. And we are all working universally for that same cause, to make that same sound, to keep that same beat, same rhythm and then to break when you are supposed to. Everyone is very excited about that. And we know that you know that song, too. So that's what makes music work so well for all of us as long as it can be used correctly.

Music can be used incorrectly . . . it can be done wrong. If the music is too loud or too low depending on their hearing abilities or disabilities . . . all these kinds of things create problems. The environment has everything to do with it. You can make it a success or a failure. You need to take into account always who you are working with and how they're relating to the environment and what is going on. Some people find it absolutely annoying.

Sometimes I'll hear music and it's the wrong kind of music and I'll kill it or change it. For example, sometimes you need to keep them focused on a task and the music is distracting, but you have to just see what's happening and just do it. I've been working with this for seventeen years, and this disease is constantly training me . . . and I move to whatever it asks of me, and that's the way it has to be. . . .

Or for instance if you took someone who was not extroverted and you called them out in a musical setting and said, "Albert, sing this song," it would be wrong. Albert does not want to sing along, he does not want to be showcased, he does not appreciate this, and you have made him uncomfortable. Chances are that after one or two times that you do this, he will avoid music altogether.

And for some people, this is not their activity, or not their activity all the time. It truly does depend on the environment. What we have to do always is read the environment and look at what is going on in it today, not yesterday. We need to look at the situation and say, "Albert does not appear from his facial expression to be enjoying the activity." So we should remove Albert from the activity and offer him another direction to go, something different to do, so he does not feel trapped in the midst of all this sound.

Sometimes they become overstimulated, and this overstimulation can cause a negative reaction, so you need to remove them from the irritating focus. Because if Albert becomes verbal, and loud and vocal, he is going to irritate someone else and it is going to create a reaction. Everybody doesn't enjoy everything, so we have to be sensitive.

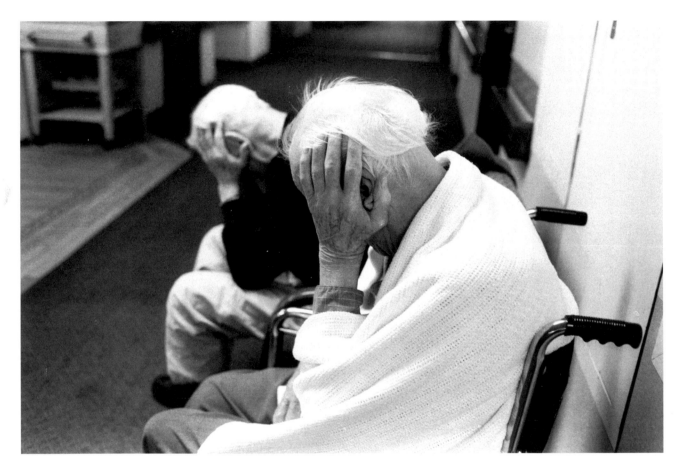

Dr. Rockwell explained that about 20 percent of people with dementia have the Lewy Body variant.
These people are sensorily overloaded. They need to be stimulated, but they can't always stand it,
so often they are happiest in their rooms. They're more autistic. It is believed that they are often actively hallucinating,
and there's so much going on in their heads that they can't deal with more.
Edgar and Glenn probably have the Lewy Body variant.

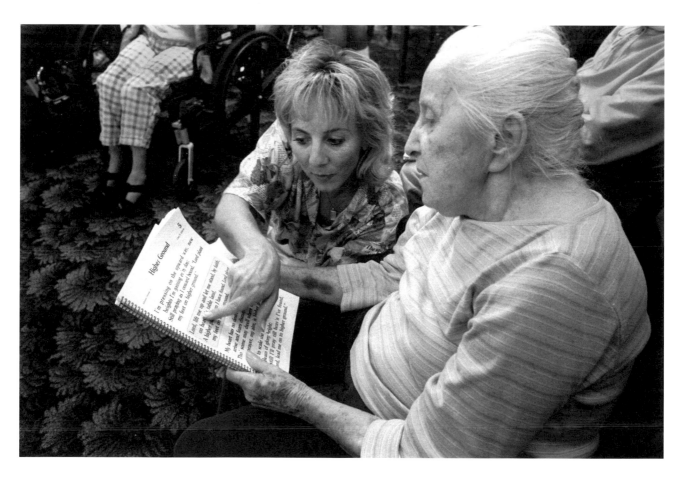

I saw residents of different faiths at religious services involving music. Almost all sang with gusto. Pat explained:

"The church comes here twice a week and they provide music at a 6:00 p.m. service. It's a Bible service,
and music is incorporated as a major part of it. It's not so much studying the Bible as it is studying religious music. . . .
That is the cornerstone. Being a Baptist and being black, it is part of my culture.
One of the first things we learn is gospel music, which has always been rich in our culture. . . .

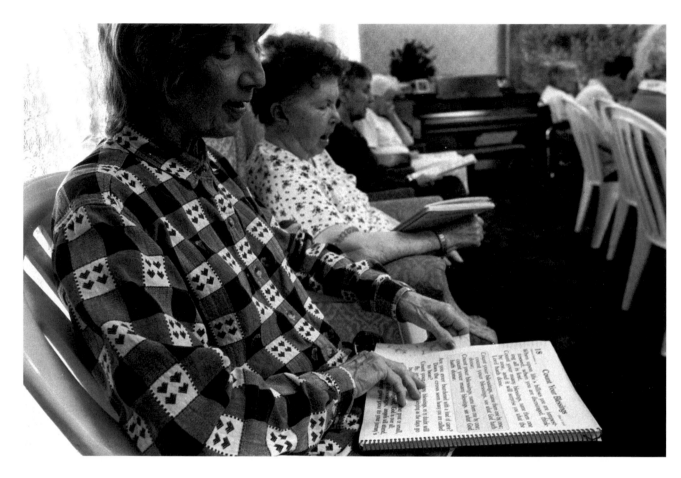

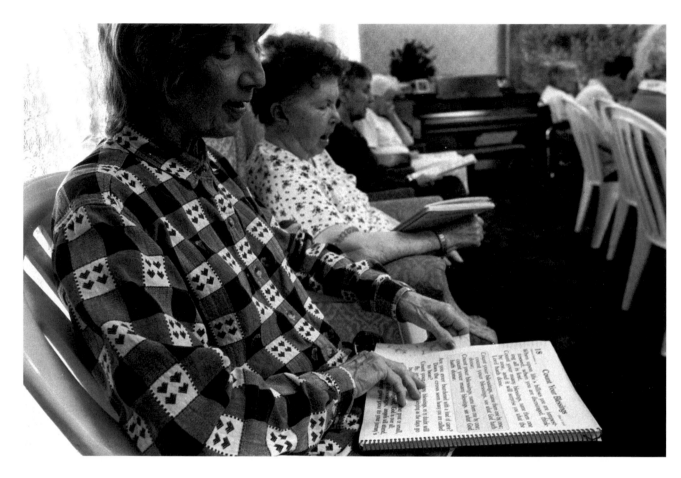

"... The ministry of music is a whole other language. When verses of the Bible don't make any sense any more,
we can use the ministry of music to give the Bible verse back in a rhythm that makes sense and never leaves you.
I can ask them to sing gospel songs and truly they are reciting the Bible with lyrics and music behind it.
And they remember it. But if I was to ask them for John 36 or whatever, they don't remember, nor would I,
for that matter. But we never forget the ministry of music. . . .

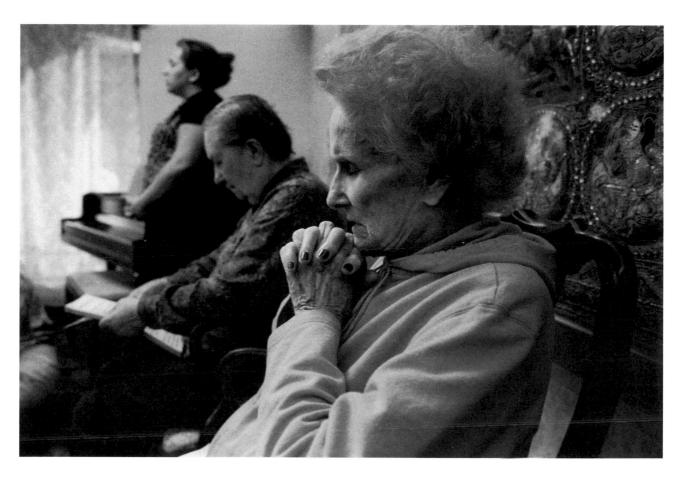

⌒∞⌒

". . . When we include music, we know that we excite them, and we keep them going. We do memory recall, and they are excited at what they can pull up and remember. So the ministry of music is extremely important."

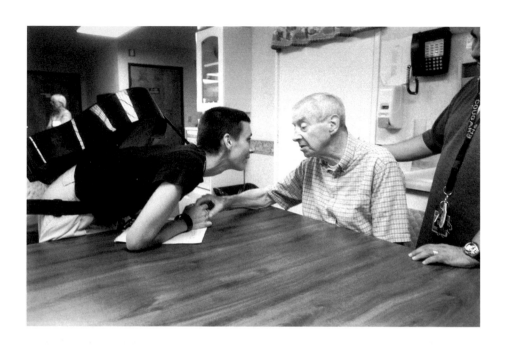

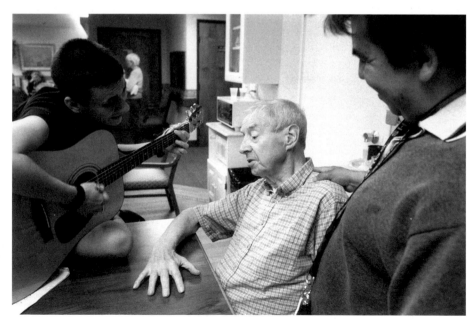

5

Waves of Remembrance

My belief in the importance of music for maintaining human connection was strengthened each Monday, from 1:00 to 8:00, when Heather, a vibrant woman in her thirties, would come to Silverado. A trained and certified music therapist, Heather started her career working with children. In 1998 a colleague who was moving out of California asked her to take over a contract involving work with dementia patients. Heather agreed, with hesitations, but she reports, "I fell into it and I loved it. I love these people. And I think I get so much from them, doing the work I do. I receive so much back from them. The gift they give me is in the form of their love, their stories, their smiles. Whatever it is that they're tapping with their foot, if they have no other way to express themselves, is such a gift for me. I love to see people express themselves through music, to see the joy that music has the ability to bring."

"Magical Mondays," I called them when I spoke of these days to my husband and my friends. As Heather moved around Silverado, some residents who were nor-

mally quiet and showed little joy lit up as soon as they saw her. Others took a few moments to recall who she was and what she did there. In each of the two large salons, Heather conducted group musical sessions, singing with the residents and singing to them. She used song books and asked each group member to select their favorite. Many residents who didn't speak clearly and logically could remember and sing all the words to such songs as "Daisy, Daisy," "Oh! Susanna," "Home on the Range." A few people always selected the same song. Others had a different basis for choice, as Heather reported was the case with Goldie: "Goldie! She makes sure to tell me every time, 'I'm 90 years old!' She will drop everything for music, when she sees me. We have this thing now, where she's told me her lucky numbers are 7 and 18, which in Hebrew means 'long life' or something. Whatever song book we're using, she'll pick the song on page 7."

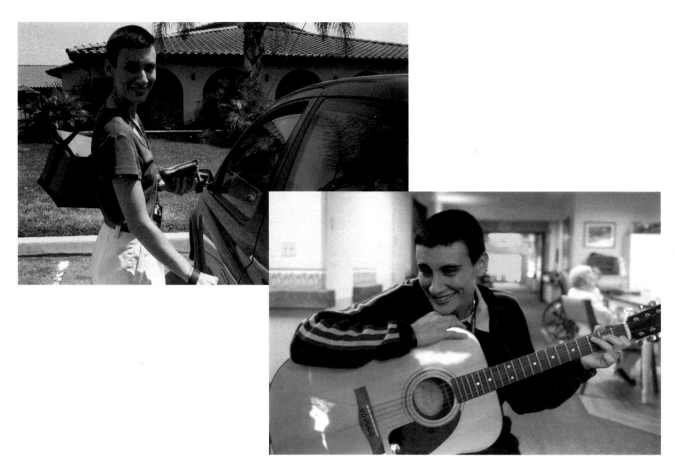

❦

"There is no amount of money that we could give Heather for what she brings to the house or what she is worth.
She has the perfect personality to work with these residents. If life ever gives Heather a bad day, she never brings it into this building,
and this is extremely important if you're dealing with dementia patients, because they are actually feeding off your emotions.
If you're not excited, if you're not happy, they seem to feel that. They sense it if you don't want them,
and they don't want you and they don't need your burden; they can't take it on."

—Pat

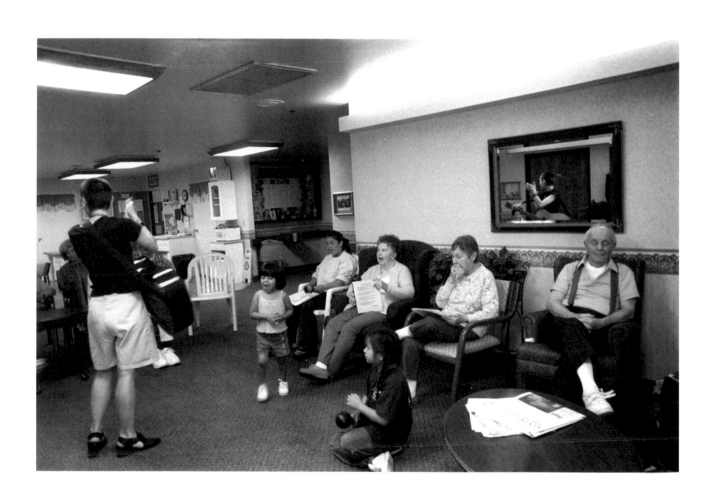

In one of our long talks, Heather described what she did and what she hoped to accomplish in the group sessions.

What I've been having people do is to make choices. Doing that taps into their long-term memory, which they get to share not only with me but a lot of times with the whole group. I've printed up some large-print song books. What I ask people to do is to scan down the cover sheet or to look through the book to make some choices about songs they enjoy, songs that they like a lot.

Often people's life stories will come out with these songs. For example, I heard a wonderful story from a woman who is now 98 who used to ride on the Wabash Cannonball, the railroad, when she was young. That's where she met her husband-to-be, riding that train! I got to hear some of her life story through her having chosen that song. It's great, it's wonderful, it's living history for me to be able to do this through music with these people.

When I'm using the song book in the group session, I'm basically using music to work on non-musical goals, including self-expression. That, of course, is part of what we're doing when we're making music: self-expression. But there are some other things I'm hoping people will do.

I'm also working on visual tracking. They scan a list of songs and choose one; now, can they scan across and identify the page? I know what page every song is on, but I will always ask, "Can you tell me what page that's on?"

Then I'm working on fine motor control, and their ability to turn pages, to manipulate pages. So we're working on their motor coordination, their hand coordination, on visualization. I'm working on the total person through music.

A lot of people feel intimidated at first; they think I'm asking them to sing the song. I always reassure them that they don't have to sing the song, but nine times out of ten they will, even if they've said, "I don't have a good voice." The song books serve as an aid to help people remember the words. A lot of times they don't know all the words, but they see them on the printed page and all these memories come flooding back.

Many times what I'll try to do is to get myself down to their eye level because I know that a lot of times people are more responsive if they're looking at me. So I'm encouraging people through just getting down to their level and singing to them, as well as to the whole group. Often they may only know some of the words, or they are just able to hum the tune, but whatever that is, I want them to be able to express that.

I also enjoy helping them engage one another when I'm doing a group session. So if one person makes a comment, or tells a story, and other people can't hear it, I might reiterate what they said, encourage other people to hear it and share their thoughts and feelings on whatever that topic was. And I want to give everyone who wants it the chance to make those choices and decisions. It's an accomplishment.

After singing, I always say, "Can you help me remember what songs we sang today? I need to write them down." What we're working on now is their short-term memory. So I write down whatever they can remember at first. Usually they have the ability to recall the last song we did. Some of them are usually able to recall five or six of the songs we did that day. Once they've exhausted their ability to recall from memory, we'll do a "Name That Tune," where I'll hum the first notes of each one. I'm asking them to figure out the name of the song from hearing the melody.

When Pat discussed Heather's effectiveness, she also stressed the importance of making choices and highlighted another of Heather's practices that incorporated this element:

> Heather has created some habits and some trends with them like the candy thing. That doesn't seem very important to most people looking at it, but it is. She has created friendships with candy. They know that after they finish singing they are all going to get candy. And everyone gets to choose out of that huge bag of candy that Heather brings in. She is allowing choices. They're dipping in and choosing what they like. She's not just giving you a Snickers bar when you don't want a Snickers bar. She's respecting their minds and giving them choices.

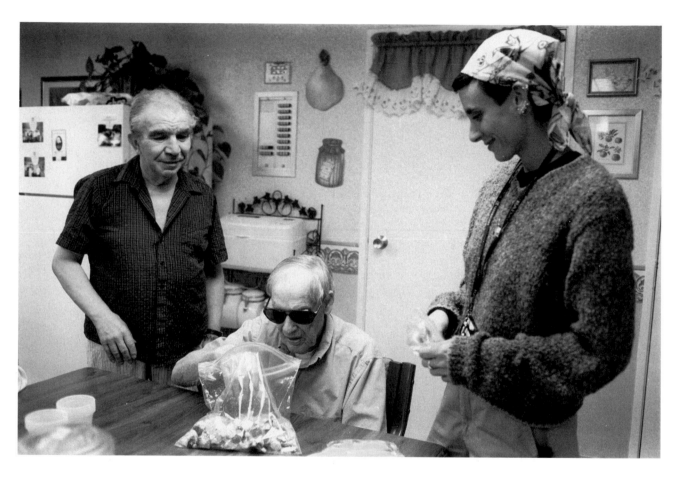

"This group suggested something to me that now I do. They suggested, 'Why don't we have a candy afterwards?'
I come from a very humanistic school of thought about music. Music in and of itself is the reward. I don't work as a behaviorist,
where if someone does a 'good job' they get a piece of candy. I always resisted that. But I thought it might be kind of
nice after singing for an hour to have some candy, so I started doing it and I've just kept doing it. And people seem to enjoy
that extra little touch afterwards. Everybody gets to choose one."
—Heather

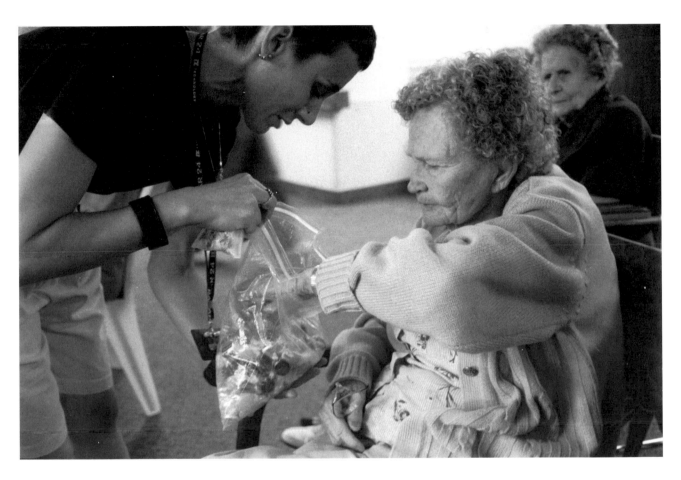

"We've been studying this. Almost all old patients, not just Alzheimer's patients, will eat candy at times that
they won't eat anything else. Part of it is that the sweet tastebuds are apparently the only tastebuds that are intact as we age.
So either you have to spice things quite a lot—but their GI systems won't tolerate that—or give them sweet things.
Most of us now know that's very important. So it's not an age reversal phenomenon, like 'They've become children.'
It seems to me that they're having so much fun, why not end with a piece of candy!"

—Enid Rockwell, M.D.

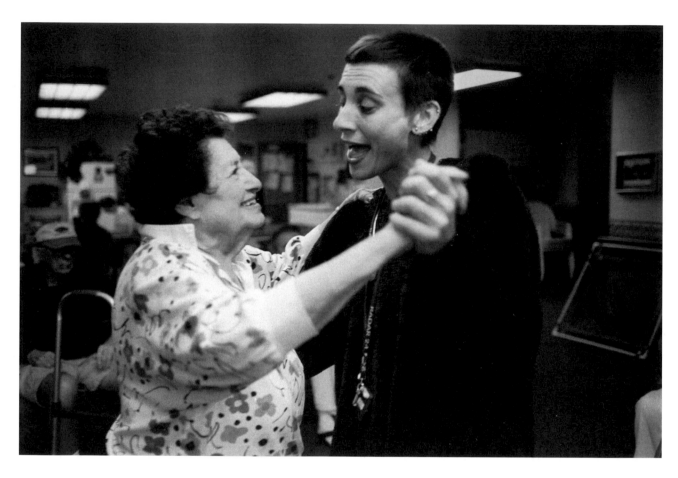

❧

"Goldie gets a kick out of the routine I do to establish stability. Every week we do the 'hello song,' then we sing from two song books, we do memory recall, we do 'Name That Tune,' I sing the 'good-bye song,' I pass out candy, and then Goldie and I dance.

"Inevitably at the end, when I collect the song books, she'll say, 'Now you're going to do "la la la"'—that's 'Name That Tune'— and 'where's my dance?' So that's our weekly routine, to have our dance together."

—Heather

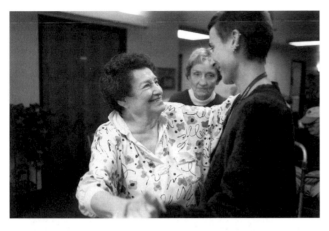

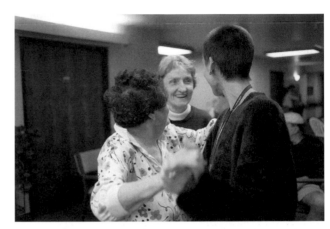

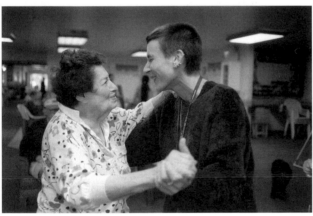

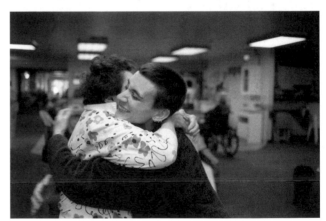

Each week, after the two group sessions with ten to twenty residents, Heather moved around the facility, occasionally working with a small group of three to four people, but mostly engaging in one-on-one interactions. Some of her work was with residents whose illness had progressed to late stages, and who related very little to other people. But in each case they responded to Heather, listened to the music, and often began to sing with her, having either selected the song or assented to a suggestion from Heather. According to Pat,

What makes it so special is that she goes to those who were not in any of the groups and she invites herself into their space and thereby invites them to her space. And they don't come into your space without an invitation. I always say God gave the Alzheimer's victim a protection, because you see that they know if you're not comfortable with them or with the environment, or if you don't like them. Heather seems to say, "My space is open to you, my ears are on you, my eyes are on you. I send my music that way. I'm happy to be here; it feels good and I feel great." If they didn't like it, they would run away and leave it and leave the music. And she would know not to follow with it. For those moments they are the star, they are in charge. And a lot of things happen: she is able to ascertain their physical ability, their vocal abilities, she can talk to them and find out where they are mentally or spiritually, she can learn things they would like to tell her about. There is a lot that goes on.

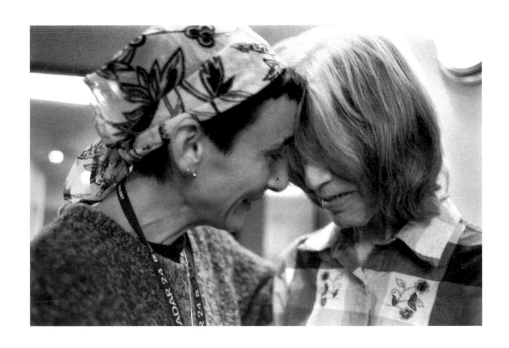

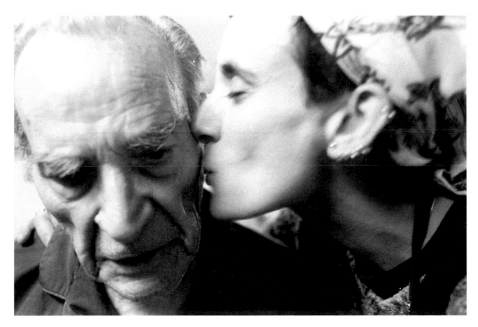

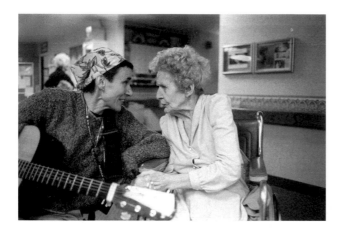
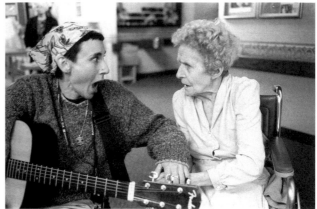

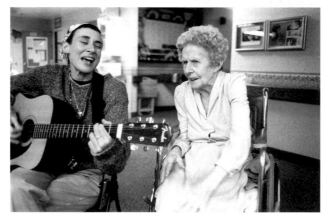

Minna and Clayton have been Dr. Rockwell's patients for several years. These photographs elicited this comment from her:

"Look at Minna! Look at the expressions! That's what they need! They need the energy and the hugging.
That's what most of them need so badly!

"You know the first thing doctors are taught is that you're not supposed to hug patients, but look!
I had a major feud at one place with the nurses, where they had taught them not to touch the patients.
I said, 'This is not a psychiatric unit, it's a geriatric unit!'"

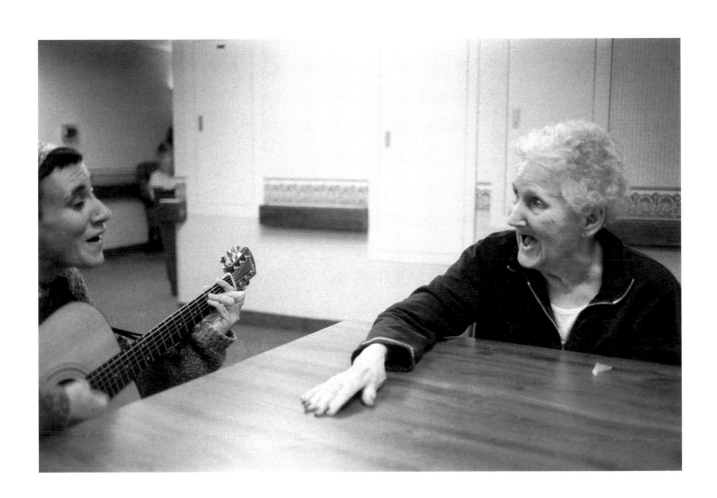

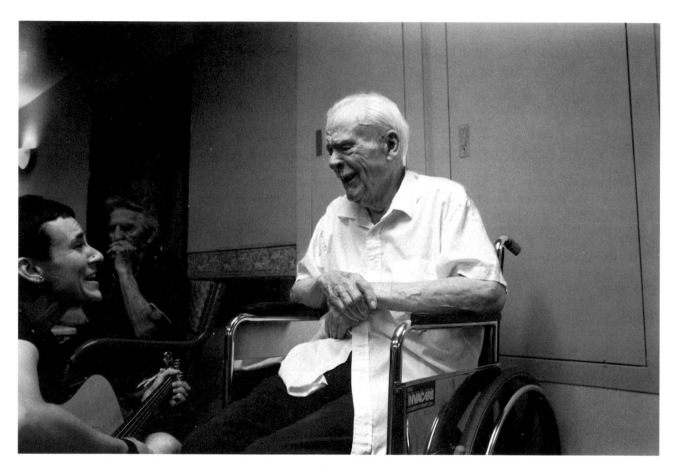

Edgar, one of the men who had their hands over their ears in an earlier photograph, sometimes liked to sing with Heather.

"This was a particularly good day. I got him at a particularly good moment. I think actually that he initiated it . . .
that I was walking by and he said something like 'Hey, give us a tune!' So that was a really wonderful experience for me,
because he's not always that engaged. But he just wanted more and more."

—Heather

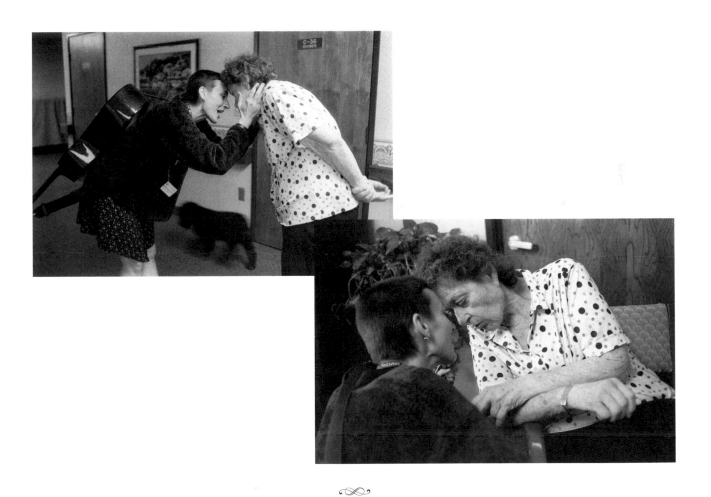

"Liz has declined a bit. She always enjoyed the music, and she was very responsive to American folk tunes like 'I've Been Workin' on the Railroad.' She would sing, with prompting. And she's such a warm, loving woman. If you walk up to her and say, 'Liz, give me a hug,' she'll just embrace you and hold you there. And sometimes it's the most healing thing for me, to get a hug from Liz. She doesn't really have the ability to talk to me anymore. But it's almost like my therapy."

—Heather

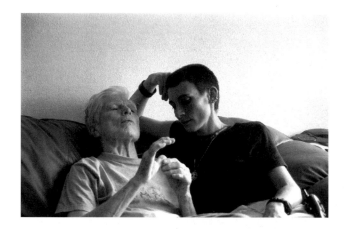
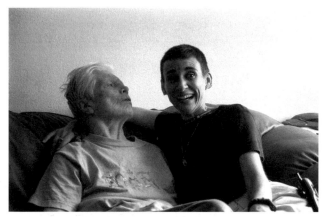
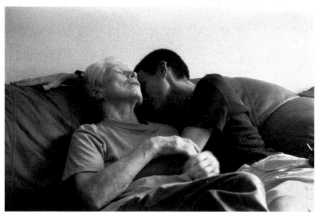

Helen was a very devout Seventh Day Adventist. When Heather started to work with her, they often walked around
the grounds of Silverado, holding hands and singing hymns. Helen couldn't take a lot of stimulation,
so Heather would sling her guitar over her back and sing *a cappella* with her. As her disease progressed,
Helen seemed to be less responsive and even sometimes aggressive when Heather sang hymns,
but she no longer had the ability to explain why. When I was there, Heather reported that Helen had become
more responsive to American folk tunes, such as "You Are My Sunshine."

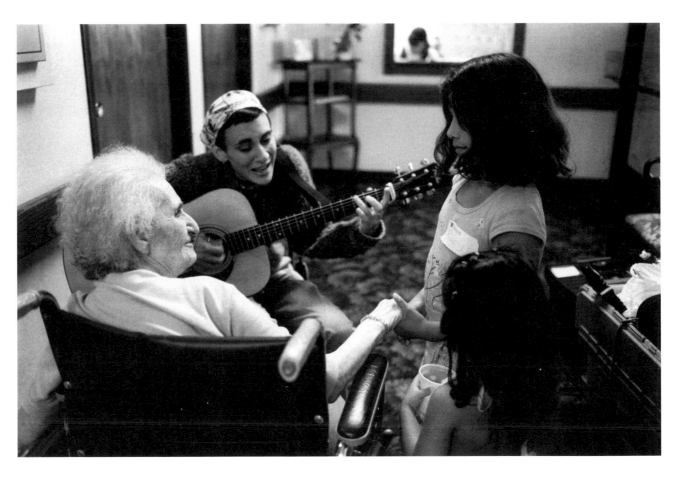

Hanna was on hospice, which means that a physician had estimated that she probably has less than six months to live. The prediction proved correct. You would not have known that watching her singing with Heather and a staff member's children. Hanna's favorite song was "The Sidewalks of New York," and she sang it with gusto.

Sue, a caregiver, had particular affection for Lars:

"Lars—this man is one of my favorites. I had him in my group for
a while, and when he sees me he always extends his hand.
Even though he can't stand up any longer and walk toward me,
he'll extend his hand and say, 'Oh my sweet . . .' Sometimes it's
hard to understand him, but you look into his eyes, his blue eyes,
and you connect. And I can tell he hasn't forgotten me.

"Lars is my Viking. That's his past history. His family were Vikings,
and he's so proud of them.
He's traveled extensively to all parts of the world.

"They've got so many stories. If we could just hear them, if they
could just tell them. We're missing so much by
their not being able to tell all their stories. You just have to take
what you can get."

Heather, too, had great affection for Lars:

"Lars and I have a special relationship. I wish you could have
been there when I was with him today.
He was more like himself today; he was reaching out and
touching my face, and talking a little more clearly.

"Lars used to be fairly high functioning, and he would wander
around the building. And while he still recognizes me now,
at that time he would become animated the minute he could
see me across the room. He taught me to say 'Thank you'
and 'You're welcome' in Swedish, and to this day when I see him,
I say those words. And he would follow me around all day long
when he was at his best. No matter where I would go, Lars was
trailing behind. He was always touching —he'd have a hand on
my shoulder or he'd hold my hand, or he'd want a hug and
a kiss. He is just a really gentle, sweet man.

"Here Lars initiated our holding hands. He kind of reached out
to the guitar, and I wanted to support that. And then he kind
of pulled back and just wanted to hold my hand. And today
that's what he wanted. So I stopped playing the guitar
and sang *a cappella*, and he sang with me. That's what's more
important, that human connection that's made through
the music."

Lars died a week later.

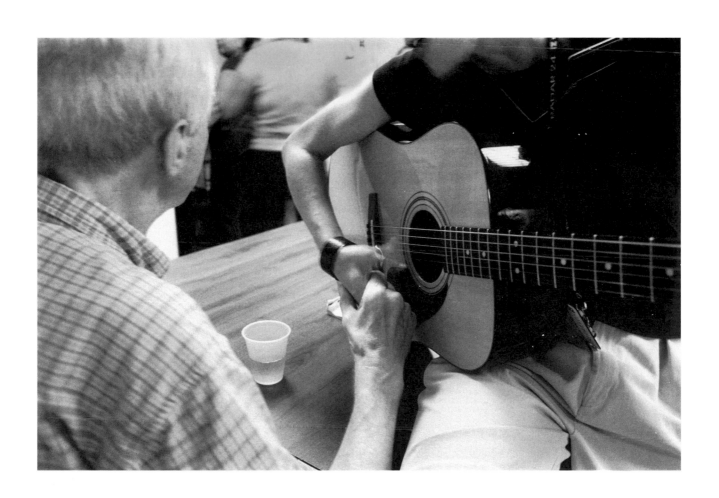

Pat commented on Heather's interactions with the residents:

Heather is not afraid of the disease. Even when residents are dying she goes to their bedside and gives them an activity. I appreciate that because when we tell our families that we are going to take care of these people to their death, they do not necessarily know what that entails. Does it mean that we are going to keep them cozy and comfortable in their beds when they are in the final stages and keep them clean and keep the sheets nice and pristine? Or does it truly mean that we go in there and act with them and talk with them and give them activities even at that time?

Heather is not afraid to do that. Early on, I told her how important I felt it was to share with them at the end. These people have been here a long time, and they pay a lot of money to be in the house, and they have employed us. So they certainly should not be left by us because they are dying. And Heather understood that and she agreed with me, and she has worked with many of the residents in the house who are on hospice. They are dying, and she goes to see them and she sings good-bye to them.

Heather and I talked about the photos of her and MaryLou that appear on pages 88–89:

I often work with people when they're dying, on hospice. The staff will call me and say, "Can you go to see so and so?" I didn't know about MaryLou until you told me you had just been with her and her daughter. I'll miss MaryLou and her stories.

The responses that I'm looking for are a relaxation in facial features, a slowing in breathing, relaxing, having people fall asleep. It's also a time for us to say good-bye when I've had a relationship with them. It's a time for me to tell them that it's OK to go, that I'll miss them, that I love them. I'll thank them for the wonderful gifts they've given me throughout the time that I've worked with them. I was probably singing "Good Journey," which is a song that I wrote. It is a song that I hope that on whatever level they can hear and understand me, that they know that they're loved.

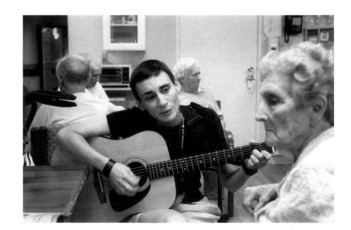

The day MaryLou stopped eating, Heather sat and sang to her.
MaryLou no longer joined in, but she listened attentively,
and the music seemed to relax her.

Good Journey

Heather Davidson (1998)

I can't remember a time
When you weren't there.
I always depended on you
And I always knew you'd care.
Now the tables have turned
And you're counting on me.
I want so much to keep you here
But I must let you go free.

At the thought that I might lose you
The spirit in me drains
But knowing if I do
For you there's no more pain.
Good journey my friend, good journey my friend
Good journey, good journey, good journey my friend.

And as I look upon your face
Expressionless your eyes
I want so much for you to stay
But I know to say, "Goodbye."
Thank you for your love
Now I offer love to you
And in the echo of my heart
I will forever miss you.

At the thought that I might lose you
The spirit in me drains
But knowing if I do
For you there's no more pain.
Good journey my friend, good journey my friend
Good journey, good journey, good journey my friend.

And as I reach out to touch you one last time
I'll take your hand and whisper
Good journey my friend, good journey my friend
Good journey, good journey, good journey my friend.

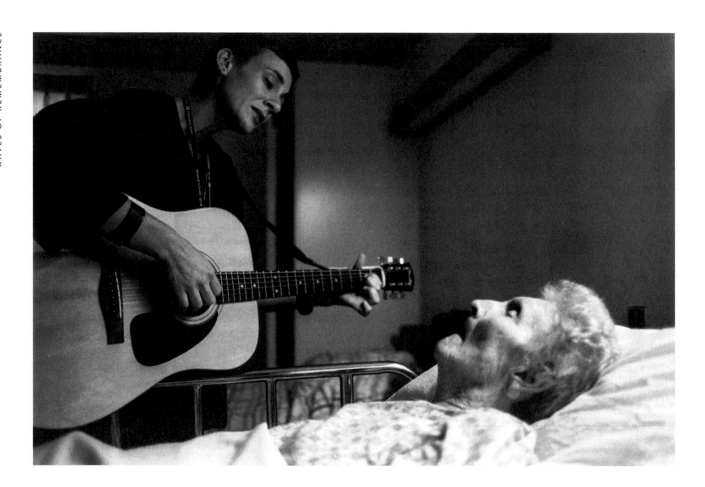

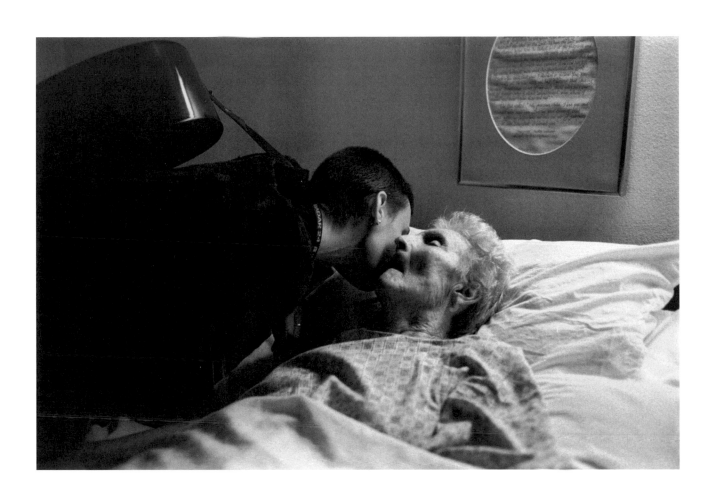

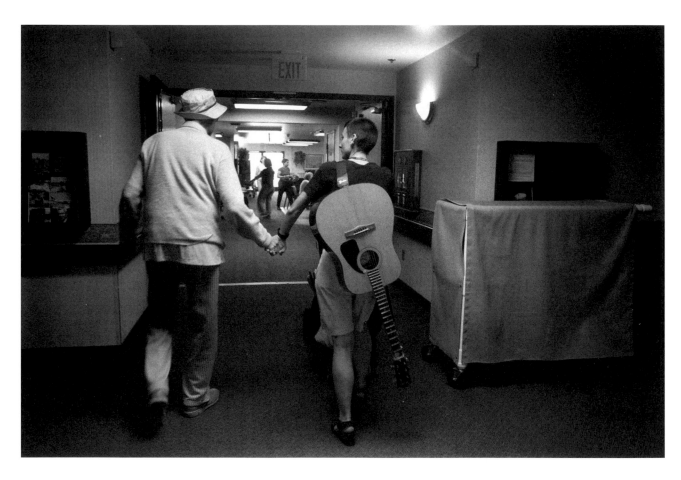

Heather welcoming a new resident.

How do we learn to die?

We live in a world that panics at this question and turns away. Other civilizations before ours looked squarely at death. They mapped the passage for both the community and the individual. They infused the fulfillment of destiny with a richness of meaning. Never perhaps have our relations with death been as barren as they are in this modern spiritual desert, in which our rush to a mere existence carries us past all sense of mystery. We do not even know that we are parching the essence of life of one of its wellsprings.

François Mitterrand, foreword to de Hennezel, *Intimate Death*

6

A Window Opening

IT HAS BEEN EIGHT MONTHS since I wrote the preceding sections of this book. I completed the first five chapters while the feel and look of Silverado were fresh in my mind. But I could not write this concluding chapter until I had a better idea of whether the photographs "spoke" to others. And if they did, I needed to understand more about the impressions they made and how the work as a whole might contribute to treatment and policy thinking, and to the fears and hopes of individuals facing Alzheimer's in their private lives.

One friend, who was very positive about the chapters, warned me: "I find it inspiring, but maybe people are too afraid of Alzheimer's to be willing to look at it, even at photographs in a book." I worried about this until several other early readers asked for a copy to show to a family member or a friend making Alzheimer's decisions for a loved one, or to show to the staff of an institution where their parent was living. These people found the volume sad, they said, because it was about a tragic disease and its toll. They found it uplifting, they said,

because it gave them hope, showing that there was another way, a better way, to think about Alzheimer's disease, those who suffer from it, and the kinds of care we give them as individuals, as professional caregivers, and as a society. The work showed (literally) that people with Alzheimer's were still very much alive and convinced them that they should be treated as such.

I then pondered the lessons I had learned from my time at Silverado. I had conversations with many old and new friends; I read the work of Nancy Mace and Peter Rabins (*The 36 Hour Day*), William Thomas (*Life Worth Living*), and Marie de Hennezel (*Intimate Death* and other titles only available in French), as well as several medical books, and memoirs written by people with Alzheimer's and by their family members. I read poignant stories on Web sites created by adoring and exhausted family members of people with the disease. Many of them had exceeded their capacities to offer home care, but had found no humane or affordable alternatives in institutional settings.

Alzheimer's, I knew, could not be seen just as an individual or a family or a medical concern. The disease is a pressing social problem, affecting millions of people, and the social costs are great. In the United States, for example, the Institute of Aging at the National Institute of Health reports the following:

AD is the most common cause of dementia among people age 65 and older. It presents a major health problem for the United States because of its enormous impact on individuals, families, the health care system, and society as a whole. Scientists estimate that up to 4 million people currently suffer with the disease, and the prevalence (the number of people with the disease at any one time) doubles every 5 years beyond age 65. It is also estimated that approximately 360,000 new cases (incidence) will occur each year and that this number will increase as the population ages.

These numbers are significant now and will become even more so in the future. Since the turn of the century, life expectancies have increased dramatically. An estimated 35 million people—13 percent of the total population of the United States—are now aged 65 and older. According to the U.S. Bureau of the Census, this percentage will accelerate rapidly beginning in 2011, when the first baby boomers reach age 65. By 2050 the number of Americans aged 65 and older will have doubled, to 70 million people.

Approximately 4 million Americans are 85 years old or older, and in most industrialized countries, this age group is one of the fastest growing segments of the population. The Bureau of the Census estimates that this group will number nearly 19 million by the year 2050; some experts who study population trends suggest that the number could be even greater. (NIA 2000)

A similar picture can be painted on a global basis, according to the same report:

This trend is not only apparent in the U.S. but also worldwide. As more and more people live longer, the number of people affected by diseases of aging, including AD, will continue to grow. For example, one study [Evans 1999] shows that nearly half of all people age 85 and older have some form of dementia.

I attended several Alzheimer's conferences; I saw films such as *Iris* and *Se souvenir des belles choses*. I met again with Dr. Rockwell and with other professionals working in various aspects of Alzheimer's disease care and research, and I talked extensively with people doing "end of life accompaniment" in France. I visited the Alzheimer's Café in Maastricht, Netherlands, a place where people with early and middle-stage Alzheimer's and their family or friends can gather in a joyous "normal" setting for chat, speakers, entertainment, crying, laughing. I also learned from the illnesses of some friends, the deaths of others, and the challenges of my mother's growing need for professional care as her Alzheimer's was diagnosed and progressed.

I am not a professional caregiver and this book is not a reference guide or a self-help book. What lessons do I think these photographs might contain, however, to help us face Alzheimer's?

As the quote from François Mitterrand at the beginning of the chapter indicates, most of us are active participants in a conspiracy of silence about death. Marie de Hennezel speaks eloquently about this:

We hide death as if it were shameful and dirty, We see in it only horror, meaninglessness, useless struggle and suffering, an intolerable scandal, whereas it is our life's culmination, its crowning moment, and what gives it both sense and worth.

It is nevertheless an immense mystery, a great question mark that we carry in our very marrow.

I know that I will die one day, although I don't know how or when. There's a place deep inside me where I know this. I know I'll have to leave the people I love, unless, of course, they leave me first.

This deepest, most private awareness is, paradoxically, what binds me to every other human being. It's why everyman's death touches me. It allows me to penetrate to the heart of the only true question: So what does my life mean?" (de Hennezel 1998, xi)

I believe that it is sad to die, and I believe that it is a tragedy to die without being treated as "alive" to the very end. That does not mean that I think we should do everything possible to prolong the duration of life. Rather, it means we need to treat a dying person as a living human being, not simply as a body that is failing, or as someone who can be dealt with in an antiseptic, impersonal manner.

I also have come to believe that our fear of death in general, not only our own eventual death, contributes to our resistance to the idea of institutional care. Many of us think of nursing homes and assisted living facilities as places for "hopeless cases" and for the "unloved," as "death worlds" for those whose families are too impoverished, economically or emotionally, to provide home care to the end. We do not think of nursing homes or assisted living residences as places to live, but as places to die. We believe that home is the best place to live and to die, and that we must provide home care until it is humanly impossible because of our own emotional and physical exhaustion, or until the worsening condition of the Alzheimer's sufferer makes it impossible to provide physical safety.

Hence we do not tell our spouses and children or our doctors that we want to be placed in institutional care unless we feel incapacitated and we fear that there is no one to care for us at home. And we do not view placing our loved ones in a residential facility as a positive step, but as a "last resort."

These views are bolstered by the history of reports (which happily are fewer than in the past) of elder abuse at some institutions, and perhaps by our own prior experiences with an institution at another time in our lives. Our personal experiences visiting nursing homes and assisted living facilities often reinforce these negative views. Some institutions look and feel and smell like death; even the better ones often appear cold, efficient, sterile, hospital-like, or regimented rather than individualized. Smiles, or at least genuine smiles, are rare. Laughter is nonexistent and sometimes considered inappropriate to the somber situation. Residents are usually calm because they are heavily medicated, and outbursts of anger are chastised. Television watching (or at least sitting in front of the television) is the primary "activity" of many residents. The places smack of the "reality" of lost connections, even when we visit a loved one to reaffirm those connections.

Silverado showed me that there is a different kind of institutional care, one that affirms life even while it serves as a last home for almost all who enter. I hope the photographs presented here convey this message, suggesting that family members may not always be the best caregivers for people with middle- and late-stage Alzheimer's, however committed and loving they may be. People with Alzheimer's need love, dignity, and respect, which are often lacking in the institutional setting. But when provided, as they are at Silverado, with a warm and attractive space to move about freely, stimulation on an ongoing basis, and the presence of children and pets, residents obtain benefits that are impossible for a "staff" of one or two family members to provide at home.

For those with Alzheimer's, a residential facility also offers the advantage of being with people who do not always see you in terms of the loss of "who you used to be." These losses are always painful, and the pain is difficult for family members to hide. Some family members will be as I was in my twenties with my grandfather, not knowing any better. I selfishly wanted him to be living in the present, in "reality," having "normal" conversations with me. But that would have meant his acknowledging his life in a sterile nursing home, bored and lonely. How much better for him that he thought he was still actively practicing law and going to baseball games! Some people are better equipped than I was to deal with these changes and with eccentric behaviors; they accept the "strange talk" or the "word salad" of people with Alzheimer's with forbearance, ingenuity, and good humor. But it is extremely difficult for family members to sustain that stance.

Professional caregivers trained in dementia care, however, can do this extraordinarily well, as I witnessed. They are skilled at managing the standard Alzheimer's problems of mood and temperament (depression, mania, excessive rage), cognition (defects in reasoning, memory, or capacity to form judgments), perception (hallucinations, disorientation, loss of sensory acuity), and volition (apathy, loss of curiosity or motivation). And with the assistance of family members, they can individualize their caring so that the resident is not depersonalized, but treated in terms of his or her past life, interests, and needs.

Silverado is unusual, but it does not have some hidden mystique. The success I witnessed is partly the result of the philosophy that pervades the institutional structure, and partly the result of putting that philosophy into concrete practices that reduce social withdrawal and depression. All caregivers can learn from the staff at Silverado. Other institutions can incorporate practices that reflect their approach to the residents: treat them as alive with Alzheimer's and they will be more fully alive.

Afterword

Fighting the Fear of Alzheimer's

Enid Rockwell, M.D., F.A.P.A

IN RECENT YEARS, around the world, there has been an increase in the number of reported cases of Alzheimer's disease, an increase in the percentage of the elderly diagnosed with Alzheimer's, and an increase in the average cost of treatment. Today Alzheimer's disease (AD) is the fourth leading cause of death in the United States. Between 5 and 11 percent of the population over the age of 65 will be afflicted. The prevalence doubles every five years from age 65; among those who live beyond 90 years, one out of every two individuals will have AD or a related dementia. Alzheimer's disease is the third most expensive disease in the United States, costing nearly 100 billion dollars a year. A low estimate of the average lifetime cost per patient is $200,000.

It is not surprising, then, that there is a high level of fear surrounding AD. Sometimes it seems that everyone we know has an aunt, an uncle, a parent, a grandparent, or a friend of the family affected by the ravages of the disease. "Am I next?" we worry.

Is it true that the threat is more real than it was in earlier times? Is there anything that can offer us a basis for hope? The answer to the first question, I believe, is both yes and no. The answer to the second is definitely yes; while there currently is no cure for Alzheimer's, medical research is proceeding at a fast pace, and early and proper diagnosis of AD makes more effective treatment possible. And as this book shows, it is possible to provide life-enhancing care to people suffering from the disease.

Why Are There So Many More Cases of Alzheimer's Disease Today?

The increase in the number of cases is in part due to better diagnosis and in part due to increased life expectancy. In the 1960s, when Cathy's grandfather was described as having "hardening of the arteries," senile dementia was considered a normal part of aging. A half-century earlier, in 1907, Alois Alzheimer autopsied a 51-year-old woman who had developed bizarre behavior and had a history of an unknown dementia disorder. His autopsy identified the "plaques and tangles" now known to be characteristic of what would later be called Alzheimer's disease, but for several decades little attention was given to the discovery. It was not until the 1960s that medical understanding of AD advanced in a significant way.

Since then, more attention has been paid to the disease, and considerable research has been undertaken. A Medline search indicates the marked increase in published articles on Alzheimer's disease in the past four decades:

Period	Number of Citations to Alzheimer's
1960–1969	43
1970–1979	400
1980–1989	5,653
1990–1999	18,734
2000–June 2003	8,911

With improved understanding of the condition came a better grasp of how many people were afflicted with a disease with an etiology, not just with "normal aging" problems. Dr. Robert Katzman published a landmark study in 1978, demonstrating that the prevalence of AD had been seriously underestimated. A Boston study followed (Evans et al. 1989), replicating the finding of a 30 to 47 percent prevalence in community dwellers over the age of 85.

In the same period, better knowledge and better treatment of other diseases helped to increase life expectancy. The resulting larger population of elderly meant a larger population of people with Alzheimer's disease. This is expected to continue, leading to high prevalence rates in the next decades (GAO 1998).

The increase in the number of cases is perhaps also due to improvements in treatment. When sufferers know that there is something that can be done for them, it is easier for them to seek help. Today those who experience symptoms are encouraged to seek early diagnosis because there are treatment options that can slow the pace of development of the major symptoms of the disease. For example, a class of drugs called cholinesterase inhibitors work to keep the levels of acetylcholine high. Acetylcholine, a chemical messenger in the brain, is important for memory and other thinking skills. Cholinesterase inhibitors are also helpful in treating vascular dementia, pseudodementia from depression, and the fog of fibromyalgia, and they are extremely helpful for treating Lewy Body dementia and Parkinson's dementia.

At present, three cholinesterase inhibitors approved by the FDA are prescribed: donepezil (Aricept), rivastigmine (Exelon), and galantamine (Reminyl). These medications were initially designed to treat memory and word-finding difficulties; the results were disappointing. Families of patients, however, reported improvement in patients' behavioral problems and improvement in their level of functioning, such as dressing, grooming, and participating in activities, when patients had previously lost those abilities. Other patients were observed to be more articulate, less depressed, less anxious, and even less confused.

There is a basis, then, for hope, for dealing with the fear surrounding Alzheimer's disease. But many people are not aware of the differences between normal changes in memory and performance, and the signs of AD. They may consider each instance of forgetting someone's name or the location of the car keys as a sign of early Alzheimer's. They also are not aware of the treatment options available for those diagnosed with Alzheimer's or another form of dementia. And they do not know what characterizes high quality care for people suffering from Alzhcimer's. These are big subjects, but some words here may be helpful in beginning to dispel the elements of fear that result from lack of knowledge.

Diagnosing Alzheimer's

What do we know about the disease and what progress have we made in treating it? How do we know who has Alzheimer's?

Normal aging involves a delay in the retrieval of names or words and increased difficulty learning, but when one forgets that they forgot, it is suggestive of AD. Alzheimer's disease is evidenced by short-term memory problems and difficulty in learning and naming objects. The hallmark of AD is "rapid forgetting" or "in one ear and out the other." Alzheimer's disease is characterized by the development of cognitive deficits, including memory deficits that cause impairments in social functioning and performance at work. Misplacing objects, loss of problem-solving abilities, loss of judgment, visual spatial problems (getting lost in familiar situations), difficulty in performing familiar tasks, a disturbance in functions such as planning, organizing and sequencing, and loss of motivation and initiation are other common symptoms that usually follow the memory and language problems. Gradually, the activities of daily living become an insurmountable chore.

Alzheimer's disease is characterized by an insidious onset and a slow progression of memory impairment and one or more of the following: a language impairment, the loss of the ability to carry out motor activities, the failure to recognize objects. The preservation of social skills in early AD is a common reason why physicians miss the signs of dementia. The personality changes of Alzheimer's disease are often unrecognized, or denied, by the patient himself or herself, while others increasingly observe a disturbing deterioration of behavior. The defensive behavior of a patient in denial of these changes, or a family that tries to hide the patient's "dreadful affliction," presents a major barrier to the identification of AD. The key to early diagnosis is a reliable informant.

A definitive diagnosis of Alzheimer's can only be established microscopically, following an autopsy, when the presence of plaques and tangles can be confirmed. I believe, however, that neuropsychological testing at an early stage is essential. Such testing not only identifies the type of dementia but also assesses the degree of impairment and the particular pattern of the dementia. This will allow the treatment team to develop specific recommendations for an appropriate living situation and activities that will stimulate but not overwhelm the individual.

The accuracy of a clinical diagnosis is 55 to 95 percent, depending on the level of expertise of the team evaluating the patient. A complete assessment includes a full physical exam, a neurological exam, and laboratory tests, such as complete blood count, chemistries, thyroid function, folate and B12 levels, urinalysis, perhaps a test of homocysteine level, and a test to rule out syphilis. A CAT scan or an MRI of the head will rule out a stroke, a tumor, hydrocephalis, and other causes of dementia; it will not aid in the diagnosis of AD, other than in ruling out other diseases. The Provider Checklist for Treating a Confused Elder offers what I consider a good program of diagnosis and recommendations.

Provider Checklist for Treating a Confused Elder

HISTORY AND PHYSICAL

- ❏ Mental Status Exam (e.g., MMSE)
- ❏ History of memory loss (e.g., sudden or gradual change, difficulty in performing familiar tasks, changes in personality or mood)
- ❏ Assessment for mental illness
- ❏ Evaluation for depression; treatment, if present
- ❏ Functional assessment of the patient including feeding, bathing, dressing, mobility, continence, ability to manage finances and medications
- ❏ Assessment for substance abuse or medication mismanagement
- ❏ Assessment for recent physical trauma (e.g., falls, head injury, abuse)

LABORATORY TESTS

Routine Lab Tests

- ❏ Complete Blood Count
- ❏ Electrolytes
- ❏ Blood Urea Nitrogen
- ❏ Creatnine
- ❏ Random Blood Sugar
- ❏ Calcium

Dementia Screening Tests

- ❏ TSH
- ❏ B12

Contingent lab tests (order only if patient's history indicates)

- ❏ Syphilis serology (MHA-TP or RPR)
- ❏ HIV
- ❏ Heavy metal

Diagnostic Tests

- ❏ MRI or CT scan only if clinically indicated (for a list of conditions, consult below listed guideline*)
- ❏ Rule out presence of delirium

SOCIAL AND SAFETY ISSUES

- ❏ Assessment of patient's driving ability; report to local health department, if unsafe
- ❏ Assessment of patient's decision-making capacity
- ❏ Discussion of Advance Directives
- ❏ Assessment of caregiver, which includes identification of primary caregiver and assessment of caregiver's capacity to manage person's needs (physically, emotionally, etc.)
- ❏ Assessment for elder abuse

REFER TO SOCIAL WORKER OR ALZHEIMER'S ASSOCIATION FOR

- ❏ Enrollment in Safe Return (an identification program for memory impaired persons)
- ❏ Information on caregiver support groups, as appropriate
- ❏ Information and education on dementia and disease course
- ❏ Referrals to adult day centers and respite services
- ❏ Information on legal and financial planning

Source: Alzheimer's Association of San Diego
* A useful diagnostic guideline is the *Clinical Practice Guideline on Early Alzheimer's Disease: Recognition and Assessment*, developed by the Agency for Health Care Research and Quality. To obtain a copy, call 1-800-358-9295.

This checklist is based in part on the California Guidelines for Alzheimer's Disease Management. To receive a copy of the guidelines, visit the Alzheimer's Association, Los Angeles's Web site, www.alzla.org, or call (323) 938-3370.

The average life expectancy after a diagnosis of AD has been established is eight to ten years. I have had patients die within a year of their initial evaluation, while others have lived more than twenty years.

Alzheimer's Disease and Other Forms of Dementia

Alzheimer's disease is the most common form of dementia (about 65 percent of the total cases), but numerous other dementias mimic it, though the presenting symptoms are somewhat different. Diagnosis is important because the treatment options depend upon the form of dementia that is found. The major other forms are briefly described here.

Lewy Body Dementia

Lewy Body dementia (LBD) is now the second most common dementia diagnosis in most countries. New neuroimaging techniques show that this form of dementia starts in a different part of the brain than that portion where Alzheimer's disease begins. The criteria that distinguish Lewy Body dementia from Alzheimer's disease include "fluctuations," from normal to almost delirious. The sufferer may be wildly confused, with a total resolution in hours. This is often misinterpreted as a "TIA"—a transient ischemic attack, or "ministroke." Mild Parkinson's symptoms may or may not be present. Gait disturbance and tremor unlike Parkinson's can also develop. LBD patients are notable for their behavioral abnormalities, as they are often driven by florid visual hallucinations and delusions which are seen early in the course of the illness long before memory becomes affected. Unlike Parkinson's disease, the visual hallucinations and delusions can be threatening, even persecutory.

It is the Lewy Body dementia patients who are often institutionalized first because their caregivers cannot deal with their disorientation and agitation. Doctors also have difficulty with these patients because they are so sensitive to tranquilizers. These patients require more acetylcholine-enhancement treatment than do the Alzheimer's patients and, indeed, there is often a robust response to the cholinesterese inhibitors.

Frontal Temporal Lobe Dementia

Frontal temporal lobe dementia is characterized by a change in personality, poor impulse control, poor judgment, and often language impairment before the onset of memory problems. Some spouses describe patients as aliens because they have become almost mute, apathetic, and robotic, with total loss of empathy. Other patients become disinhibited, gluttonous, disheveled, and, at times, antisocial, obsessive-compulsive, or both. Almost all frontal temporal lobe dementia sufferers lack insight into their illness. Again, an early diagnosis allows more effective treatment. These patients do not respond as well to the cholinesterese inhibitors, but they require mood stabilizers for their lability of mood and stimulants for their apathy and poor motivations.

Frontal temporal lobe dementia constitutes 5 percent of all dementias and has been the subject of recent scholarly meetings and caregiver meetings because its pathology is so unique.

Vascular Dementia

Vascular dementia can present with a stroke that produces significant motor and cognitive impairment, or it can develop in a stepwise fashion as small strokes occur.

There is also a form that can have an insidious onset and gradual development, like Alzheimer's disease.

Thanks to the efforts of modern progressive medicine, many people now exercise and watch their blood pressure and cholesterol levels, and the prevalence of vascular dementia is lower than ever before (5 percent of all dementia cases). Arrhythmias (irregular heart rates) can lead to a showering of clots to the brain, but they can be well controlled today using Coumadin (a prescription blood thinner) and other anticoagulation medications.

Parkinson's Dementia

Parkinson's dementia occurs in 40 to 60 percent of patients diagnosed with Parkinson's disease. The movement disorder usually precedes the dementia; with advanced age the likelihood of developing dementia is greater. The first sign is a slowing of mental power and an increase in forgetfulness, in contrast to the dense short-term memory impairment characteristic of Alzheimer's disease. Executive functions (planning, organization, problem solving) are lost early in the course of this dementia.

Combination Dementias

To distinguish between vascular dementia and Alzheimer's disease, medical professionals look at risk factors, such as diabetes, stroke, hypertension, and hypercholesterolemia; however, we realize that Alzheimer's disease and vascular disease often coexist, just as AD and Lewy Body dementia can coexist. The combination dementias are more lethal in that the course is more aggressive and the symptoms are more florid and treatment resistant.

The prevalence of the Lewy Body and Parkinson's dementia combination is about 7 percent; the prevalence of the Alzheimer's disease and Lewy Body dementia combination is about 5 percent; the prevalence of the vascular dementia and Alzheimer's disease combination is about 10 percent.

Treatment of Alzheimer's Disease

It has been said that the only way to prevent Alzheimer's disease is to choose the right parents. We have learned that by increasing the brain's reserve, the clinical presentation of AD can be modified. Exercise, learning, increased socialization, and a healthy diet, in addition to protecting the brain from injury, all increase the brain's reserve. The most compelling research focuses on arresting or slowing the progress of the disease.

The treatment of anxiety, depression, hallucinations, and other behavioral disorders will alleviate the most painful aspect of dementia for the patient and for the caregivers. Depression can cause a reversible dementia. When depression coexists with AD or other dementias it aggravates both the symptoms and the course of the disease. Given the reversible aspect of this dementia, aggressive steps must be taken to control the symptoms. The patient's quality of life can improve markedly even if there is an underlying dementia, uncovered after the depression is treated.

Anxiety alone or associated with depression occurs in almost every Alzheimer's patient during the course of the illness. Agitations become more prevalent as the disease progresses. Anxiety is very toxic to the areas involved in memory and will cause more pronounced atrophy of the hippocampus and adjacent structures in the brain. Thus treatment should be directed to the reduction of anxiety.

Effective treatment does not mean just medication. In 1984 Dr. George Glenner discovered the sequencing of Beta amyloid. Realizing how important it was to create activities that maximize the existing skills of the patient, especially socialization, he and his wife, Joy, went on to open the first Alzheimer's family day care program. They also knew that the caregivers were suffering and needed support and education. For many, a day care program provides both stimulation for the Alzheimer's patient and respite for the family caregivers. If the newly diagnosed patient stays at home without activities, they will deteriorate more rapidly. The treatment for this disease is stimulation and socialization, which is more therapeutically powerful than any medication we can employ at this time.

Dementia patients need to be stimulated seven days a week. They need to have just the right amount of activity. You cannot throw them into a family reunion because their symptoms will escalate from overstimulation. This is a fine balance, and it cannot be achieved for the majority of patients at home. Some day care programs, however, do a tremendous job.

For those at later stages of their illness, some residential programs also do great work, as this book has so well demonstrated. Alzheimer's sufferers at a later stage of their illness continue to require stimulation but also have additional needs that are often beyond the abilities of family members to provide adequately. If quality institutional care is available and affordable, it is often the best choice for both patients and family members.

Forms of Institutional Care

Long-term care facilities are divided into three categories: (1) nursing homes; (2) domiciliary care residencies; and (3) Hospice. In the United States, these forms differ in terms of what they provide, how they are staffed, and how they may be paid for by various forms of insurance.

Nursing Homes

Nursing homes are either skilled nursing facilities, or SNFs (pronounced "sniffs") or intermediate care facilities. The SNF provides twenty-four-hour nursing care. Medicare will only reimburse for the period necessary to stabilize a patient requiring acute medical intervention, roughly two weeks. The Medicaid patient will be covered in many SNFs; however, Alzheimer's special care programs often require private payment. The advantage to living at a SNF is that there are federal regulations that are strictly enforced. Medications must be reviewed by the doctor every month to ensure that they are helpful. If a patient is doing well, the reviewers will suggest lowering the dose or stopping the medication. Should the staff feel that the drug is necessary, the doctor will need to write a rationale for continuing it. Other facilities do not have such a rigorous audit. In some types of residential programs, a social worker will perform the review. Intermediate care facilities provide care for patients with less serious medical problems. They do not routinely accept Medicare. Long-term care policies will reimburse part of the cost. Nursing home care costs vary by geographic location, and generally range between $2,500 and $10,500 per month, with a national average of $4,654 per month, putting it beyond the means of most people.

Domiciliary Care Residences

Domiciliary care residences, otherwise known as rest homes, homes for the aged, or custodial care homes, are not medically oriented, but they do provide supervision for patients with chronic medical or mental illness. Neither Medicare nor Medicaid will reimburse this level of care, but SSI will provide supplemental funds for qualified individuals.

The assisted living facility is a relatively new version of residential care that was first instituted to provide a transition from independent living to SNF care. Assisted living facilities offer meals and a range of activities; many focus on patients with dementia. The more expensive facilities usually offer a more creative environment and activities from morning to night and on weekends, but there are exceptions. Families lured by a lower cost at assisted living facilities often do not realize that the dementia patient will not be able to survive long in a setting that is not specially designed for them. Silverado is an example of an assisted living facility specifically tailored to the needs of people with dementia, and that is one key to its success with the people shown in this book.

Unfortunately, assisted living centers are not covered by insurance policies, except some long-term care policies. The rates average $2,500 to $5,000+ per month. The better programs have a higher level of nursing supervision and often an R.N., twenty-four hours per day. This is a critical point. Only an L.V.N. or R.N. is able to assess for "as needed" medications. At the assisted living level, the M.D. must fax an order if the medication schedule is to be altered in any way.

Multilevel facilities include independent assisted living and SNF care. One may enter at any level, but only the residents who came as "full-level care" will be assured of having a place at the higher levels of care when it becomes necessary. This can be a costly endeavor—the entrance fee is quite high, in addition to monthly fees of $1,000 to $3,000. A multilevel facility can be ideal, however, for the individual who wants total security. Usually only a portion of the entrance fee is refundable, and in some communities it becomes nonrefundable after five years. Recently, these often glamorous communities have included Alzheimer's special care units.

Facilities known as board and care homes are often operated by charitable or nonprofit organizations. They provide twenty-four-hour supervision, meals, and some personal assistance. In the smaller homes, activities are generally marginal because the facilities are "mom and pop" operations. The cost is substantially less; however, the medical supervision can be problematic. On rare occasion, the limited staff will have been trained. The more successful homes establish a relationship with a physician team that makes house visits.

Other specially designed housing for elder care includes foster care and elder cottage housing opportunity, or ECHO, better known as "granny flats." My objections to dementia patients living in a private home under foster care are the lack of stimulation, the absence of peer interaction, and the increased risk for accidents, unless the patients are going to Alzheimer day care. The caregiver will eventually burn out, and the situation sometimes becomes abusive. ECHO housing has been quite successful for non-dementia care; the associated social services agency attempts to match an adult with an older individual in need of an informal companion. This is not an option for a person with a dementia illness, however, because the renters are not skilled caregivers and they are not supposed to be responsible for any personal care.

Hospice

Hospice is now becoming involved in Alzheimer's special care programs and has offered their expertise to overextended staff and the family system of the patients. The power of Hospice is both their humane treatment of the terminal patient with regard to pain and their ability to help the families to cope with the impending loss. They also work with the special care staff and assist them in the grieving process that a devoted caregiver experiences. They provide group therapy and individual counseling, and they attempt to reach the dementia patient through nonverbal communication. Most health insurance covers this specialized Hospice care, which averages one to six months or more in SNFs. The Hospice hospital unit cannot accommodate a patient for than a few weeks and is generally not designed for Alzheimer's patients.

Life-Enhancing Alzheimer's Care

Differences in care are not just decorative. The right approach can create care that is indeed life enhancing. Unfortunately, this is not typical. Peter J. Strauss and Nancy M. Lederman describe the situation all too accurately:

> Even with recent improvements, nursing homes by nature are impersonal places, designed to offer production-line, albeit humane, services marketed to the least common denominator.
>
> We say this not by way of criticism, but to remind you that personal contact, caring, and interest are qualities that are hard to measure but very important for you to consider. A facility that has compassionate staff, that manages to engage its residents in activities of interest to them, that establishes some sense of warmth in individual quarters and common rooms— these are things that cannot be quantified but that will be invaluable, literally life-saving, to residents. (1996, p. 36)

One of my first rotations in geriatrics was at a prestigious long-term care facility. I will never forget the display of Chagall paintings or the Rolls Royces at the entrance. I will also never forget the stark rooms and the patients who confided in me that they were threatened not to call the nurses at night. They were instead instructed to urinate or defecate in their diapers and told that they would have to remain in that state until the morning shift arrived.

When I came to San Diego in 1985, I was astounded by two small SNF Alzheimer's special care facilities tucked away in the periphery of the county. The exterior of each was unimpressive, but the moment I opened the door, the love and the warmth enveloped me. There was a sense of peace and contentment (not drug induced) among the patients, the staff, and the families. The families were encouraged to come as often as they wanted. I had never experienced the power of incorporating the family into the environment in such an intimate manner. Dogs, cats, and pomegranate trees ripe with fruit lay hidden behind the modest architecture of the home. This skilled nursing facility turned out to be one of the precursors to the first Silverado. One of the secrets to Silverado's success is the fact that the original administrator of the two precursor facilities continues to head the staff as new branches are opened.

Silverado is an excellent example of an "enriched environment" specially tailored for the dementia patient. The majority of patients will never need to move to a higher level of care, given the strong emphasis placed on mobility and the efforts of an enthusiastic staff. Creating the "enriched environment" involves having enough activities to stimulate the brain to create more connections or synapses and to sprout new neurons. Avoiding overstimulation is equally important because it will lead to agitation.

Also critical is having a high level of nursing care to evaluate for pain, infection, adverse effects of medications. Unless there is a pharmacist available or at least a

Certified Nurse Assistant, grave mistakes can occur. For example, many assisted living centers use "bubble pack" medications so that a low-level caregiver can dispense them. In these cases, the supervision is not adequate. These aides do not know why the patient is receiving a certain medication or what side effects to look for. At Silverado, a staff nurse provides this attention to medications.

The real strength of an Alzheimer's special care program rests on its foundation, the nursing supervisor and aides. The best programs have strong supervisors who provide hands-on training. The staff must also be of sufficient number to give patients one-on-one attention when necessary. To create the ideal environment, it is critical that aides have experience with behaviorally disturbed dementia patients. The aides must be dedicated caregivers, speak English, and articulate clearly to be able to communicate with the patients and their families. The patients can sense when a caregiver is angry or frustrated, cold, or indifferent. They will often react with agitation. In return, these caregivers must be reimbursed appropriately. The facility administration and the family must acknowledge and celebrate the sacrifices the caregivers make and reward them for their empathy and their hard work. They must be treated with respect. Unfortunately, too many programs focus on cosmetics and skimp on wages, offering as little as $6.50 per hour. This practice will lead to a rapid turnover of staff. The consistency, reliability, and security vital to creating the appropriate environment cannot be maintained under these conditions.

In sum, in the best environments the staff must do several important things:

- Obtain an understanding of the prior lifestyle of the resident in order to maintain his or her identity and dignity. The staff must be aware of the resident's past educational background, career, level of activity, coping styles, and level of comfort with socialization.
- Do not expect the patient to remember the date or the location of his or her room. Some of the better facilities mask doorways or eliminate them altogether to avoid having the patients feel locked up and to prevent disorientation. Others use color coding to help provide orientation. "Memory boxes," such as those in use at Silverado, help residents to find their own rooms and help staff to remember the particular history and prior achievements of the resident.
- Know how to assess for pain, hunger, wetting, or soiling. Most patients are not reliable historians; they have lost the ability to articulate their feelings and to self-report somatic symptoms. When questioned, they may deny pain, especially when it is intermittent. Many dementia patients never receive analgesics despite the fact that their charts document arthritis. This omission has been a recent focus in the management of dementia.
- Anticipate and modify situations that provoke anxiety. Alzheimer's patients can exhibit tremendous anger and frustration over their feelings of loss of control and abandonment. Should caregivers react in a defensive or punitive fashion, they will only precipitate an escalation in the disturbing behavior.
- Follow a written routine. Consistency, structure, and sequencing are therapeutic for the AD patient because the disease strips them of the ability to plan, organize, and learn new and different material.
- Understand that communication with the AD patient requires simple sentences, conveying one idea at a time. Speaking slowly, repeating, avoiding shouting, and using nonverbal cues such as a nod and a smile when possible is recommended. Confrontation is

never an acceptable mode of communication. Correcting the patient is also discouraged. Whenever this is observed at home or in a residential facility, it should be identified and modified; the dementia patient is not a child.

- Understand clearly the several established triggers that will produce anxiety, fear, or agitation. Overstimulation, fatigue, or excessive demands will usually end in the development of a behavioral problem. A change in the environment or caregiver will be problematic. Even a change in routine can have grave repercussions. Large groups, ill-behaved children, and elaborate decorations that hide the cues that patients use to navigate have been cited as forms of overstimulation. Misinterpretations of television programs can occur because of how the Alzheimer's patient's brain functions (for example, one patient threw a pail of water on two men fighting on TV to get them to stop; another would not speak to his wife because she would not feed the stranger in the mirror).

- Know that stimulation is essential to life enhancement. This is not only a question providing activities. Understimulation can also occur when an activity is not satisfying to a patient.

This list is, of course, incomplete, but it is suggestive of the facets of a program that can make an institutional placement a most positive experience, not a "last resort."

Fighting Fear through a Deeper Understanding of What Remains after Alzheimer's

This book shows the results of high quality, life-enhancing care. The photographs demonstrate that these residents are alive far beyond what is generally believed by the general public and even by many physicians with years of experience with Alzheimer's patients. I had visited Silverado many times, listened to the positive reports of family members of my patients and other residents living there, made rounds there and in many other facilities, and had been greatly appreciative of their efforts and successes before I introduced Cathy to the site. Nonetheless, I was astounded when she began to show me her photographs. I saw evidence here of a capacity to thrive, to enjoy a quality of life, to respond to stimuli, far beyond what practitioners usually see, focused as we often are on the problematic side of the illness. We are often so far from knowing about this kind of interaction of our patients.

These photographs are extraordinary for practitioners, for family members, for everyone to see what's going on with these people. The stimulation pictured in this book is more powerful than any medication that we will have in our lifetime. These photographs can sensitize everyone to what is possible in Alzheimer's care. They so vividly show us that there are people inside these bodies, people with personalities, who experience emotion, and they show that there is life after Alzheimer's. Given this society's fear of aging, and the frightening statistics on Alzheimer's disease, people can't help but fear the worst. In these pages readers will see that it is a disease, and it does destroy parts of people; they are not who they were before in many ways. But readers will also see that these people are still alive, that there are still wonderful things that come from them and that can be done to maintain their dignity and integrity and joy.

References

Evans, D. A., et al. Prevalence of Alzheimer's Disease in a Community Population of Older Persons: Higher Than Previously Reported. *Journal of the American*

Medical Association 262 (1989): 2551–56.

GAO (General Accounting Office). 1998. *Alzheimer's Disease: Estimates of Prevalence in the United States.* Report to the Secretary of Health and Human Services, GAO/HEHS-98-16. Washington, DC: U.S. General Accounting Office.

Katzman, Robert, Robert D. Terry, and Katherine L. Blick, eds. 1978. *Alzheimer's Disease: Senile Dementia and Related Disorders.* New York: Raven.

About the Author

Enid Rockwell is a Distinguished Fellow of the American Psychiatric Association (F.A.P.A.). At the University of California San Diego Thornton Hospital, she is the medical director of the Senior Behavioral Research Program, chief psychiatrist for the Seniors Only Program, and consultant to the Alzheimer's Research Center. She is also an associate clinical professor of geropsychiatry at the UCSD Medical School.

Silverado Senior Living was founded in June 1997 by Loren Shook, CEO; Jim Smith, CFO, and Steve Winner, Chief of Culture. Since its inception, the mission has been to give life to those whom others have given up on. Steve Winner often explains that the three wanted to create a community that was an alternative to spending the rest of one's life in a nursing home, in a medical environment.

Corporate Offices

Silverado Senior Living—Corporate Office
27121 Calle Arroyo, Suite 2220
San Juan Capistrano, CA 92675
Telephone: (949) 240-7200
Fax: (949) 240-7270

Facility Locations

There are currently twelve Silverados: four in Texas, one in Utah, and seven in California. Information on each of these facilities is available from the corporate offices, or on the Web at www.silveradoseniorliving.com. Visitors from around the world are regularly welcomed to see for themselves how the philosophy is put into action, how the mission is achieved.

The Silverado facility you have just seen and read about is in Escondido, California. The director is Kathy Greene.

Silverado Senior Living—Escondido
1500 Borden Road
Escondido, CA 92026
Telephone: (760) 737-7900
General Fax: (760) 737-8184
Nurses Fax: (760) 735-6707

Technique

These photographs were taken with a Canon EOS Elan camera, using 28 and 35 mm lenses. Kodak Tri-X film was used without flash. The negatives were scanned with a Nikon Super Coolscan 8000. Final images were made with Photoshop 6.0 and imported into a QuarkXPress document. None of the images have been cropped.

Alzheimer's and Aging

Aldridge, David, ed. 2000. *Music Therapy in Dementia Care.* London: Jessica Kingsley.

Barnett, Elizabeth. 2000. *Including the Person with Dementia in Designing and Delivering Care: "I Need to Be Me!"* London: Jessica Kingsley.

Braff, Sandy, and Mary Rose Olenik. 2003. *Staying Connected While Letting Go: The Paradox of Alzheimer's Caregiving.* New York: M. Evans.

Cheston, R., and M. Bender. 1999. *Understanding Dementia.* London: Jessica Kingsley.

Hennezel, Marie de. 1998. *Intimate Death: How the Dying Teach Us How to Live.* New York: Vintage Books.

Fazio, S., D. Seman, and J. Stansell. 1999. *Rethinking Alzheimer's Care.* Baltimore, MD: Health Professions Press.

Hudson, Rosalie, ed. 2003. *Dementia Nursing: A Guide to Practice.* Ascot Vale, Victoria, Australia: Ausmed Publications.

Ignatieff, Michael. 1994. *Scar Tissue.* New York: Farrar Straus & Giroux.

Judd, Stephen, Mary Marshall, and Peter Phippen, eds. 1998. *Design for Dementia.* London: Hawker.

Killick, J., and K. Allan. 2001. *Communication and the Care of People with Dementia.* Buckingham: Open University Press.

Mace, Nancy, and Peter V. Rabins. 1999. *The 36-Hour Day.* 3d ed. Baltimore, MD: Johns Hopkins Press.

Marshall, M. ed. 1997. *State of the Art in Dementia Care.* London: Centre for Policy on Ageing.

Patel, Nina, Naheed R. Mirza, Peter Lindblad, Omar Samaoli, and Mary Marshall. 1998. *Dementia and Minority Ethnic Older People: Managing Care in the UK, Denmark, and France.* London: Russell House.

Peterson, Ronald, ed. 2002. *Mayo Clinic on Alzheimer's Disease.* New York: Kensington.

Shenk, David. 2001. *The Forgetting: Alzheimer's—Portrait of an Epidemic.* New York: Doubleday.

Snyder, Lisa. 2000. *Speaking Our Minds: Personal Reflections from Individuals with Alzheimer's.* New York: W. H. Freeman.

Strauss, Claudia J. 2002. *Talking to Alzheimer's: Simple Ways to Connect When You Visit with a Family Member or Friend.* Oakland, CA: New Harbinger.

Strauss, Peter J., Nancy M. Lederman, and Kjell J. Espmark. 2003. *The Senior Survival Guide: Everything You Need to Know to Safeguard Your Money, Health, and Freedom.* New York: Facts on File.

Thomas, W. H. 1996. *Life Worth Living : How Someone You Love Can Still Enjoy Life in a Nursing Home: The Eden Alternative in Action.* Acton, MA: VanderWyk & Burnham.

Zgola, J. M. 1999. *Care That Works: A Relationship Approach to Persons with Dementia.* Baltimore, MD: Johns Hopkins University Press.

Visual Sociology/Documentary Photography

Becker, Howard. 1986. Do photographs tell the truth? In *Doing Things Together*, 273–92. Evanston, IL: Northwestern University Press.

Bot, Marrie. 1988. *Bezwaard Bestaan*. Rotterdam: Marrie Bot.

Emmison, M., and P. Smith. 2000. *Researching the Visual*. Thousand Oaks, CA: Sage.

Franck, Martine. 1980. *Le temps de vieillir*. Paris: Editions Denoël-Filipacchi.

Gold, Steven. 1989. Ethical issues in visual field work. In G. Blank, James McCartney, and Edward Brent, *New Technology in Sociology*, 99–109. New Brunswick, NJ: Transaction.

Harper, Douglass. 1988. Visual sociology: Expanding sociological vision. *American Sociologist*, Spring, 54–70.

Harper, Douglass. 1994. On the authority of the image: Visual methods at the crossroads. In *Handbook of Qualitative Research*, ed. N. K. Denzin and Y. S. Yvonna Lincoln, 403–12. Thousand Oaks, CA: Sage.

Hevey, David. 1992. *The Creatures Time Forgot: Photography and Disability Imagery*. New York: Routledge.

Jury, Dan, and Mark Jury. 1976. *Gramp*. New York: Grossman.

Mark, Mary Ellen. 1990. *The Photo Essay*. Washington, DC: Smithsonian.

Markisz, Susan, 2001. You don't win a Pulitzer by accident. *The Digital Journalist*. http://digitaljournalist.org/issue0109/star_intro.htm

Ohm, Karin Becker. 1977. What you see is what you get: Dorothea Lange and Ansel Adams at Manzanar. *Journalism History* 4 (1):14–22, 32.

Papademas, Diane, ed. 2002. *Visual Sociology*. Vol. 2. Washington, DC: American Sociological Association.

Rainey, Matt, and Robin Gary Fisher, 2000. After the fire. *Newark Star Ledger*. Weeklong series at http://www.nj.com/specialprojects/index.ssf?/specialprojects/afterthefire/main.html

Smith, W. E., and A. Smith. 1975. *Minamata*. New York: Holt, Rinehart & Winston.

Spence, Jo. 1988. *Putting Myself in the Picture: A Personal, Political, and Photographic Autobiography*. Seattle: Real Comet.

Watney, Simon. 1987, Photography and AIDS. *Ten-8* No. 26: 14–29.

Alzheimer's Organizations and Services

The following Web addresses are provided as additional resources; however, any questions regarding a medical diagnosis, treatment, referral, drug availability, or pricing should be directed to either a licensed physician or to the product's manufacturer.

Alzheimer's Association (USA), www.alz.org

ADEAR: Alzheimer's Disease, Education and Reference Center, National Institute of Aging (NIA), www.alzheimers.org

Alzheimer Europe, www.alzheimer-europe.org

American Association for Geriatric Psychiatry, www.aagpgpa.org

The Cognitive Neurology and Alzheimer's Disease Center, www.brain.nwu.edu

Doctor's Guide, www.docguide.com

The Mayo Clinic offers a very useful set of guidelines for considering a long-term care facility. Print out the set of questions in their section on "Long-term care options" under Alzheimer's Disease and take it with you when you make visits: http://www.mayoclinic.com/invoke.cfm?objectid=EEBBC4A3-9361-44DC-8AB176322039E59C

One's first encounter with someone afflicted with Alzheimer's can result in many different responses but the first are usually fear, frustration, anger, impotence, regret, and the desire to flee the specter of loss. It is only later, and not always for everyone, that a renewed sense of intimacy, connection, and thankfulness are established. My first experience with Alzheimer's was in the person of my grandfather. I had all the negative feelings, but I never got to the positive states with him. I did learn from our encounters that I needed to live my life as fully as health and luck permitted. I also took as a lesson that it was not always good to "leave the best for last." So I begin the acknowledgments of my debts for this project with the "best," with the person usually cited last, the partner who supported and endured the long process of preparing this book. My husband, John Gagnon, inspired this project even before its inception. I had taken a long break from photographic work, feeling that I was not doing it as well or as frequently as I wanted. For several years John persisted in encouraging, pushing, prodding a return to my camera and darkroom. He also encouraged the laser eye surgery that allowed me to stop complaining about the way the glasses I had needed since my early forties banged into the camera. He fostered all my efforts to rekindle my enthusiasm and build my photographic confidence. Once I had started working again, he endured endless interruptions as I showed him images, told him stories of my days' adventures, discussed my frustrations and insights, and repeatedly sought his advice. Later he helped me select images for exhibitions and for the book, reviewed text, and offered insight on everything. Mostly he kept me remembering, as he does in the rest of my life, what is important. Thank you, John.

Now, back to the beginnings.

It was in a master class from Mary Ellen Mark that I began to work on a project on the aged. I would not have selected the site she assigned for my photographic work during the course, the Asilo Municipal de Santa Rosa, because I was afraid of old-age homes. But I was also afraid to tell Mary Ellen about being afraid! Through my initial time at the Asilo and through a subsequent trip to expand my photographs and interviews, I discovered that I could not only tolerate this environment, but that I could learn and grow, indeed even thrive, from the relationships I built with the residents. The class also changed my photographic approach and helped build my confidence as a photographer. I had long admired Mary Ellen's work, and her guidance and encouragement to build on

ACKNOWLEDGMENTS

my initial work with her was critical to my continuing to the Silverado project. Marcella Taboada, a talented Mexican photographer who served as Mary Ellen's local contact person during the course, also provided friendship and encouragement during both my stays in Oaxaca.

Seeking a site to photograph the aged during the summer of 2001, I asked everyone I knew in the La Jolla area for assistance. My friend Dr. David McWhirter, a San Diego psychiatrist, introduced me to his colleague Dr. Enid Rockwell, a geriatric psychiatrist at UCSD Medical School and Thornton Hospital. Enid invited me to join her at one of the family support group sessions she ran monthly at the Escondido Silverado facility, telling me she thought it was a cutting-edge place for people living with Alzheimer's. She introduced me to the staff there and later met with me to review my photographs and help me to understand what in them was important. I can think of no one more appropriate to write the afterword for this volume, and I am grateful to her for agreeing to do so.

At Silverado I received an extraordinary welcome. Kathy Greene, director of the facility, provided constant assistance, information, and support for my efforts, from the first day to the day the final draft of the manuscript was completed. I cannot begin to thank her sufficiently for the open door and the open heart she provided.

Tracey Truscott, the social worker at Silverado, and Renee Hamilton, then in charge of family relations, were also warm and welcoming throughout my stay. Along with Kathy, Tracey was instrumental in securing the final permissions from family members for the photographs used here. The contributions Pat Thompson made to my understanding of the themes of this project are evident throughout the book. And the Mondays I spent watching Heather Davidson work enriched my life, as well as my stock of photographs and my appreciation of the power of music. I continued to benefit from ongoing communications with her as I prepared the manuscript.

The rest of the Silverado staff also made me feel always welcome. Their smiles, their conversations, and their sharing of their views of what was transpiring in my photographs made my work pleasurable and boosted my understanding of the site and my appreciation of the spirit that still resided in the residents. Many family members and friends of the residents also helped, and I thank them all. Ken Fussel, in particular, guided me to a better understanding of the impact of Alzheimer's on spouses, and to the rewards of placing a loved one in a facility like Silverado.

Before I had a book project in mind, discussions of my photographs with several friends persuaded me that others would learn something about Alzheimer's from seeing this work. Encouragement from Bennett Berger, Chandra Mukerjee, Joe Gusfield, Irma Gusfield, Mary Walshok, Garry Shirts, and Cozette Shirts led me to begin to prepare exhibition materials. Dan Stein visited me in California and went to see Silverado for himself, as the photographs showed him a quality of care he had never seen through his years of medical practice. His enthusiasm helped reassure me I was on to something important.

A half-hour meeting scheduled with an old friend and colleague, Doug Harper, turned into a three-hour discussion, followed up in many e-mail messages and phone conversations. Doug offered invaluable help in both the sociological and photographic interpretation of my work. I hope he sees the results of his advice in this final product. Feedback from students in my visual sociology class and my graduate-level qualitative methods class at Rutgers University in the fall of 2001 was also of great help. Particular thanks are due to Miriam Moscovici, Maria Islas, and Brad Crownover. Barry Haynes taught me about digital printing and Wendy Crumpler encouraged me to create a book from the prints during a week spent with them in Oregon.

Two Rutgers colleagues were extraordinarily helpful. Julio Nazario's years of experience as a photographer and as a photography teacher at New York's International Center of Photography gave me much needed assistance in the process of selecting the best images from the hundreds I had taken. Ferris Olin's years of organizing art exhibitions and her knowledge of the art world were coupled with her friendship and generosity; she assisted me at many stages of preparation of the manuscript and provided many concrete ideas for exhibition and publication.

Winning a prize in the French national photographic competition, FNAC Talent 2002, for a dossier of twenty of these photographs bolstered my confidence greatly and convinced me that the photographs "spoke" to people about new ways of thinking about Alzheimer's. I am indebted to the anonymous judges of that competition, to the organizing committee of the European Alzheimer's Society's 2002 meeting, and to Amelie Codafy Brétonnière at FNAC Nice for inviting me to exhibit a portion of this work. The many people who offered their thoughts on the exhibits at these venues also contributed to my understanding of what are the important messages in this work. Special thanks are needed for Sandrine Lavalle, the communication officer at Alzheimer Europe. Enthusiasm for the photographs from Bernadette Keene and Cynthea Wellings at Ausmed Publications when I met them at the Frankfurt Book Fair was also much appreciated. They requested use of the photograph of Stacey, Roxy, and Dorothy (page 29) for the cover of one of their Australian company's many excellent books on dementia, and Cynthea visited Silverado during a trip to the United States as a response to seeing the first draft of this book. I also owe thanks to John Hollander, for permission to reprint his "Poem Sent on a Sheet of Paper with a Heart Shape Cut Out of the Middle of It," from *The Night Mirror*, copyright © 1971 by John Hollander.

A number of close friends read various drafts of the manuscript and offered their suggestions; all were keen readers, and some of them shared stories of their own family struggles with finding good Alzheimer's care. Many thanks to Philippe Moussier, Judy Mengin, Nicky Isaacson, Dennis Meadows, Suzanne Meadows, Leslie Greenblat, Kevin Greenblat, André Hankard, Colette Hankard, Vivian Satori, Luc Schuhmacher, Katherine Schuhmacher, Kristelle Lanzi, Elisabeth Guillerm, Saburo Kimura, Kiyoshi Arai, Stuart Katz, Alexandre Gaillard, Françoise Bisson, André Chenet, Jocelyn Cha, Jean-Claude LaPorte, Jean-Marie Panzini, Brigitte Panzini, David Crookall, Ellye Bloom, and Yves Loureau.

Responding to my quest to bring this book to a wider audience, several people have offered their expertise and their assistance, particularly Enid Rockwell, Liz Schwartz, Phyllis Lessin, and Sally Jesse Raphael. I appreciate their input greatly and I know I will continue to benefit from their expertise. Chris Cory's advice on many matters has been full of intelligence and insight. His regular e-mail messages have offered me invaluable ideas presented with wit and warmth. I am grateful for his friendship and his assistance.

And of course in the last several months I have benefited from the extraordinary work of various people at the University of Chicago Press. Douglas Mitchell, Senior Editor at the Press, first learned of this project in August 2001 as I was finishing the photographic work at Silverado. He looked at a small set of work prints, which had been neither organized, framed, nor contextualized. But he "got it," he understood the message about Alzheimer's care to be conveyed, and over the next ten months he expressed keen interest in seeing a rough draft of the

ACKNOWLEDGMENTS

manuscript as soon it was finished. I repeatedly explained that I wanted to create a document that would reflect my background as a sociologist, but that would speak, largely through the photographs, to a larger, more general audience of people who were concerned about Alzheimer's and care of people with Alzheimer's. Perhaps UCP was therefore not the right publisher, I protested, talking to other publishers who had also expressed interest. Doug persisted in his explanations of why Chicago could do the best job with this book. His enthusiasm, erudition, and energy won me over. As he sang the praises of the manuscript I gave him, and ushered it so effectively through the process of approval, I realized the value of having an editor who offered such an unwavering commitment to the project and such a good understanding of it. Now, many months later, my belief in those qualities has been more than sustained, and Doug has earned my deep and enduring appreciation.

My e-mail folder titled "UCP team correspondence" offers superb testimony to the efforts of the wonderful people at the University of Chicago Press who turned the mocked-up manuscript I sent them into a "real" book. Tim McGovern worked doggedly on the hundreds of tasks that are essential to all books, but particularly to one with photographs, permissions, and essential input from various people. Russell Harper and Jenni Fry polished the manuscript; Ryan Li used his design skills to make a book with the "feel" I had indicated I wanted, but with a professional look. Siobhan Drummond's behind-the-scenes production efforts made everything move smoothly. Erin Hogan has already offered advice in response to my many inquiries, far ahead of the scheduled time for her skills to be brought to the tasks of publicizing the book. All these wonderful people made me feel the production of the book was a true partnership, not one in which the author had to step to the side and let the editorial team take over. They allowed me to remain engaged in the decision-making and the creative thinking, and they gave their sound advice on a continual basis, always with good spirit, as I asked hundreds of questions. Most importantly, at all stages I found that this was a team that was excited about the book, about its message, about the impact it could have on thinking about Alzheimer's care.

Nice, France
October 2003